30 Days to Beat Type 2 Diabetes Naturally

Break Free from the Chains of Diabetes with this Comprehensive Action Plan

Brenda F. Dozier

Table of content

Introduction

It is during the quiet hours of self-reflection, when life takes an unexpected turn and presents us with a diagnosis, that the journey toward taking control of our lives begins. When it comes to the obstacles that are associated with health, receiving a diagnosis of type 2 diabetes can be particularly intimidating since it brings about shadows of uncertainty and change. On the other hand, hidden among these shadows is an opportunity—the possibility to rewrite the story of one's health and well-being.

You are welcomed with open arms to begin on the life-altering journey that is waiting for you during the following thirty days. This is not merely a guide; rather, it is a compass that points in the direction of a life independent of the limitations imposed by type 2 diabetes. This message extends an invitation to go on a journey of self-discovery, comprehension, and empowerment.

At the same time that you are holding this guide in your hands, you are standing on the precipice of change. This is a defining moment in which the choice to take charge of your health will echo with important implications. The following is not merely a collection of words; rather, it is a guided roadmap that has been meticulously constructed to lead you through the complex landscape of reclaiming your life from the grips of diabetes.

In the following chapters, we will decode the complexities of type 2 diabetes and provide you with a thorough action plan. We will also unravel the layers of type 2 diabetes. Every day is a fresh chance for personal development and transformation, ranging from the fundamental comprehension of your diagnosis to the practical tactics for meal planning, physical activity, and overall well-being with a holistic perspective.

This is not a journey you need to do alone. Through the tales in these chapters, the advice offered by healthcare professionals, and the support of a community committed to change, you will discover the companionship needed to travel this journey. This guide is more than knowledge; it is a companion on your journey to well-being.

So, let us go on this journey together as we manage the hurdles, celebrate wins, and move ahead toward a future when Type 2 diabetes is not a constraint but a conquered chapter in the story of your life—the power to break free lies inside you, waiting to be awakened each day. Your journey begins today.

Understanding Type 2 Diabetes

Understanding Type 2 Diabetes entails peeling back the layers of a complex health disease that has become increasingly prevalent in our society. At its core, Type 2 Diabetes is a metabolic ailment characterized by insulin resistance, a condition where the body's cells become less receptive to the insulin it generates. Insulin, a hormone generated by the pancreas, is vital for controlling blood sugar levels by enabling the absorption of glucose into cells for energy.

As we go into the physiological underpinnings, it's crucial to know that genetics, lifestyle choices, and environmental effects contribute to the development of Type 2 Diabetes. While a genetic predisposition may heighten the risk, lifestyle decisions such as food, physical activity, and overall health have a key impact.

The narrative of Type 2 Diabetes is often interwoven with the rise of obesity. Excess body weight, particularly around the belly, is associated with insulin resistance. The complicated dance of genetics and lifestyle unveils a significant role in the formation of this illness.

Blood sugar regulation, a delicate equilibrium, becomes broken in Type 2 Diabetes. When insulin fails to shuttle glucose into cells effectively, blood sugar levels climb, causing a range of health hazards. Over time, the pancreas may fail to produce sufficient insulin, leading to a progressive degradation of the body's ability to manage glucose.

Understanding the relevance of glycemic control is crucial. Elevated blood sugar levels, if left mismanaged, can lead to a cascade of consequences. From cardiovascular concerns to renal problems and nerve damage, the impact of uncontrolled Type 2 Diabetes is far-reaching.

However, the narrative need not be one of gloom. Through knowledge, lifestyle improvements, and proactive health management, individuals can recover control. Empowerment rests in grasping the varied nature of Type 2 Diabetes, recognizing its triggers, and embracing a holistic approach to health that extends beyond the prescription pad.

In the chapters that are to follow, we will unravel the practical methods and insights essential to traverse this landscape, empowering you to take responsibility for your health and rewrite the story of Type 2 Diabetes. The journey toward understanding begins with a solid comprehension of the condition's complexity – a knowledge base upon which we will create concrete steps toward a healthy, diabetes-free

future.

What is Type 2 Diabetes?

Type 2 Diabetes stands as a prevalent health concern, a metabolic illness marked by changes in the body's ability to manage blood sugar levels properly. At its core, the development of Type 2 Diabetes is closely related to insulin resistance, a disease where the body's cells become less receptive to the insulin generated by the pancreas. This important hormone performs a vital function in promoting the absorption of glucose into cells for energy, maintaining a delicate balance within the bloodstream.

Genetics, lifestyle variables, and environmental influences provide the dynamic backdrop against which Type 2 Diabetes unfolds. While a genetic predisposition may enhance the risk, lifestyle decisions like as food, physical activity, and overall health are key influences. The narrative typically intertwines with the rising tide of obesity, when excess body weight, particularly around the belly, becomes a crucial player in the formation of insulin resistance.

The complicated balance of these elements results in a disturbed dance of blood sugar management. Elevated glucose levels become a hallmark of Type 2 Diabetes, providing a range of health hazards if left untreated. The gradual nature of the illness might strain the pancreas, eventually limiting its ability to produce sufficient insulin, and further increasing the difficulty of glucose regulation.

Understanding the relevance of glycemic control is crucial. Unmanaged high blood sugar levels represent a risk for multiple consequences, compromising cardiovascular health, kidney function, and nerve integrity. The narrative, however, need not be one of gloom. Education and proactive health management empower individuals to recover control.

To comprehend Type 2 Diabetes, it is vital to recognize that this ailment extends beyond a solitary moment in time. Rather, it is a dynamic process controlled by a combination of hereditary variables and lifestyle decisions. By unraveling the layers of Type 2 Diabetes, individuals can empower themselves with the knowledge needed to traverse this health terrain, making educated decisions and embracing a holistic approach to health. This core understanding serves as a cornerstone for the actionable steps and tactics that follow, paving the road for a healthier, diabetes-free future.

The Impact of Diabetes on Health

The impact of diabetes on health is a diverse and widespread worry that extends well beyond the immediate challenges of managing blood sugar levels. Type 2 Diabetes, in particular, can throw a wide-ranging shadow on several elements of an individual's well-being.

One of the key battlegrounds is cardiovascular health. Diabetes considerably enhances the risk of heart disease and stroke. The complicated dance between increased blood sugar levels and the vascular system sets the setting for a cascade of events that can lead to arterial damage, atherosclerosis, and eventually, cardiovascular problems.

The kidneys, too, endure the load of diabetes. Uncontrolled high blood sugar levels can overtax these important organs, leading to diabetic nephropathy. Over time, this condition may lead to chronic kidney disease, further underlining the systemic impact of diabetes on the body.

Neuropathy, a disorder affecting the nerves, is another dimension of diabetes's influence on health. Individuals with diabetes may suffer tingling, numbness, or discomfort, particularly in the extremities. The peripheral nerves become prone to injury, impairing sensory perception and general nerve function.

The eyes, sensitive to variations in blood sugar levels, are also vulnerable. Diabetes increases the risk of illnesses such as diabetic retinopathy, which can lead to vision impairment or even blindness if left untreated. Regular eye examinations are critical for detecting and managing these potential issues.

Moreover, diabetes can damage the body's immune system, leaving individuals more susceptible to infections. Chronic inflammation, a typical companion of diabetes, can exacerbate current health concerns and bring extra obstacles to general well-being.

Beyond the physiological burden, the mental and emotional toll of diabetes should not be overlooked. The difficulties of managing a chronic condition, necessary lifestyle adaptations, and the awareness of potential problems can add to stress and worry, influencing mental health.

Understanding the far-reaching impacts of diabetes on health highlights the need for proactive management and lifestyle adjustments. It is a cry to arms, pushing individuals to prioritize their well-being, engage in regular health monitoring, and embrace a holistic approach that addresses the physical, mental, and emotional elements of living with diabetes. By doing so, individuals can lessen the burden of diabetes and develop a foundation for a healthier and more resilient future.

Importance of Taking Control

The value of taking control in the area of Type 2 Diabetes cannot be emphasized. It surpasses the everyday monitoring of blood sugar levels; it is an empowered posture that can change the direction of one's health and well-being. In a situation where the collaboration of circumstances can influence the course of the disease, the decision to take control becomes a linchpin for a better future.

Central to this drive is the idea that diabetes is not only a spectator sport. It demands active participation and engagement. The obligation to monitor blood sugar levels, make intelligent dietary choices, and engage in regular physical activity rests firmly on the person. This is not a passive journey; it's a proactive posture towards wellness.

Taking control extends beyond the physical sphere to the mental and emotional domains. It involves establishing a mindset that views diabetes not as an insurmountable problem, but as a challenge to be overcome with fortitude and tenacity. Embracing this perspective enables individuals to negotiate the emotional terrain that often accompanies chronic diseases, supporting mental well-being.

The ripple effect of taking control is visible in the prevention and management of diabetes-related problems. By aggressively regulating blood sugar levels, keeping to prescribed prescriptions, and maintaining a healthy lifestyle, individuals can decrease the chances of cardiovascular disorders, kidney problems, and nerve damage. The proactive strategy offers a barrier against the potential implications of uncontrolled diabetes.

Furthermore, the decision to take charge represents a commitment to a holistic strategy. It is an understanding that health is a sum of its aspects - physical, mental, and emotional. Lifestyle adjustments covering nutrition, exercise, and stress management help not only glycemic control but to an overall enhancement of well-being.

Taking control is an expression of agency in the face of a health crisis. It is a declaration that diabetes does not define, but rather, catalyzes positive transformation. Through informed decision-making, active engagement, and a dedication to comprehensive health care, individuals can carve a route toward a future where diabetes is not a restriction but a conquered chapter in the narrative of their lives. The relevance resides not simply in the act of control, but in the transforming potential it contains for a healthier and more empowered living.

Chapter 1

Foundations of a Diabetes-Free Lifestyle

Establishing the foundations of a lifestyle free from the limits of Type 2 Diabetes demands a thoughtful and informed approach. This initial phase acts as the bedrock upon which the journey towards better health is formed. As we begin this exploration, the first crucial step is to decipher the subtleties of the diagnosis and, in doing so, create a foundation built on understanding and acceptance.

In the opening days of this journey, grasping the complex nature of one's diabetes diagnosis is paramount. This is not only a label but a guidepost to understanding how the body handles glucose and insulin. It's a foundation created via education, demystifying the terminology and concepts related to diabetes. Armed with this knowledge, individuals can begin to establish a connection between the nuances of their physiology and the lifestyle choices that affect their health.

Simultaneously, the creation of a support system represents a vital component of the foundational phase. Family, friends, and healthcare professionals become pillars upon which individuals lean for advice, encouragement, and understanding. Establishing open lines of communication with these critical support networks produces a climate conducive to informed decision-making and sustained motivation.

This early phase is a time to create a positive mindset, recognizing the potential for growth amid the challenges provided by diabetes.

Embracing the diagnosis as a call to action rather than a deterrent is key to designing a lifestyle that surpasses the constraints of the ailment. It is a mindset that respects the power of choice and sets the stage for the transforming journey ahead.

In setting the foundations for a diabetes-free lifestyle, individuals engage on a path of self-discovery and empowerment.

This is a phase of education, connection, and mentality cultivation — the building blocks of a lifestyle that not only manages diabetes but transcends it.

Through understanding, support, and a positive mindset, the framework is laid for the actionable tasks and strategies that will develop in the next days of this transforming journey.

The Diagnosis Decoded

The Diagnosis Decoded stands as the cornerstone of knowing and navigating the complicated terrain of Type 2 Diabetes. This important moment, marked by the disclosure of a diabetes diagnosis, needs a comprehensive decoding of the complexities inherent in this health condition.

At its root, the diagnosis discloses the body's struggle with insulin resistance—a crucial hallmark of Type 2 Diabetes. Insulin, a hormone generated by the pancreas, serves as the key that unlocks cells, allowing glucose to enter and provide energy. However, in the diabetic setting, this mechanism finds resistance. The body's cells become less receptive to insulin, resulting in higher blood sugar levels.

Understanding the diagnosis extends beyond a mere admission of elevated blood sugar levels; it includes looking into the elements that lead to this metabolic imbalance. Genetic predisposition, lifestyle decisions, and environmental circumstances converge to define the landscape of diabetes. It is a mosaic where each component, when interpreted, provides insight into the voyage ahead.

Decoding the diagnosis is not a single endeavor. It is a joint endeavor involving healthcare professionals, individuals, and their support systems. In this time, clear and open contact with healthcare providers becomes crucial. It is through this discourse that individuals obtain insights about their distinct diabetic profile—knowledge that provides the compass for navigating the route to a healthy future.

The decoding process is not without its emotional undertones. Acceptance, frequently a crucial part of the journey, entails coming to terms with the reality of the diagnosis. It is a transforming step that lays the way for proactive decision-making, lifestyle adjustments, and the cultivation of a good mindset.

The Diagnosis Decoded serves as a template for the voyage ahead. It is the starting point for education, self-awareness, and the construction of a path towards optimal health. By learning the nuances of Type 2 Diabetes, individuals can begin to untangle the complexity, obtaining the knowledge and empowerment needed to design a road toward a life that transcends the restrictions of the diagnosis.

Grasping Your Diabetes Diagnosis

Grasping the reality of a diabetes diagnosis is a key point in one's health journey, involving a sophisticated knowledge that goes beyond the mere recognition of raised blood sugar levels. This phase entails navigating through the layers of information, emotions, and adaptations that come with the awareness of a chronic condition.

The first step in grasping the diagnosis is to realize the consequences of insulin resistance—the primary characteristic of Type 2 Diabetes. Insulin, the hormone responsible for enabling the entry of glucose into cells, faces resistance in this scenario. Cells become less sensitive, leading to a buildup of glucose in the bloodstream. This foundational understanding sets the stage for future decisions and activities in managing the disease.

Beyond the physiological element, recognizing the diagnosis includes acknowledging the role of numerous contributing factors. Genetic predisposition, lifestyle choices, and environmental circumstances converge to shape the diabetic landscape. Each component, when analyzed, provides vital insights into the specific context of an individual's health, laying the foundation for individualized interventions.

Engaging with healthcare providers becomes an important element of this phase. Clear communication and a willingness to seek help are crucial to knowing the nuances of one's diabetes profile. This coordinated effort ensures that individuals have the information and assistance needed to make educated decisions regarding their health.

Emotionally, grasping the diagnosis includes a process of acceptance—an acknowledgment that paves the way for proactive efforts toward optimal health. It's about knowing that a diabetes diagnosis is not a verdict but a starting point for education, self-awareness, and lifestyle improvements.

Grasping your diabetes diagnosis also includes grasping the dynamic interaction between genetic variables and lifestyle decisions. The mosaic of contributors generates a unique pattern for each individual, underlining the customized aspect of diabetes care. This knowledge underlines the value of adapting tactics to address specific areas of one's health, providing a sense of autonomy and control.

This period of understanding necessitates a proactive approach to instruction. Learning about the complexity of blood sugar management, the role of insulin, and the impact of lifestyle on diabetes empowers individuals to make informed decisions. It converts the diagnosis from a mystery disease into an understandable world that individuals can explore comfortably.

Engaging with a healthcare team gives not only medical expertise but also a partnership in controlling the condition. The joint effort entails setting realistic goals, addressing treatment choices, and developing a structure for continuous support. It is via this cooperation that individuals can comprehend the subtleties of their diagnosis and build a path for their health journey.

Embracing the emotional element of the diagnosis needs more than just acceptance; it is about resilience and a positive outlook. Acknowledging the hurdles while maintaining an optimistic mindset develops a mental landscape suitable for sustained lifestyle adjustments. It is an awareness that every modest step towards well-being is a success in the face of hardship.

In the area of health, information is empowerment. Grasping the diabetes diagnosis is about more than just grasping medical jargon; it is a path toward self-awareness and informed decision-making. By navigating this period with a blend of understanding, teamwork, and emotional resilience, individuals create the framework for a future where diabetes is not a barrier but a driver for good change.

Overcoming the Initial Shock

Confronting the initial shock of a diabetes diagnosis is a key period that involves emotional toughness and adaptability. The disclosure of a chronic ailment can be an unexpected and stressful experience, generating a variety of feelings ranging from astonishment to dread. In this phase, overcoming the initial shock becomes a key component of forging a route toward a balanced and empowered response.

Understanding the diagnosis is typically accompanied by a wave of emotions, and it's reasonable to feel a sense of incredulity or even denial. However, identifying these emotions is the first step toward overcoming the shock. It is a process of self-compassion, knowing that managing a diagnosis is not only a physical journey but an emotional one as well.

Engaging in open and honest conversations with healthcare providers plays a critical role in this process. Establishing a discourse regarding worries, anxieties, and questions provides a platform for getting guidance and reassurance. Healthcare experts become partners in navigating this unfamiliar region, offering insights and techniques that help pave the way for a smoother adjustment to the new reality.

Overcoming the initial shock is also about reframing perspectives. Rather than viewing the diagnosis as a constraint, individuals can choose to consider it as a stimulus for good transformation. This adjustment in mentality involves realizing that the trip ahead, albeit tough, is a chance for personal growth and a renewed dedication to general well-being.

Building a support system becomes an invaluable tool during this era. Sharing the diagnosis with close friends and family develops a network of encouragement and understanding. In these interactions, individuals find not just emotional support but also practical guidance in enacting lifestyle changes and navigating the daily obstacles of managing diabetes.

Additionally, seeking help from community resources and online forums can create a sense of camaraderie. Understanding that others have experienced similar obstacles and have successfully adapted to living with diabetes can be a source of inspiration and encouragement.

Overcoming the initial shock is a process of resilience and adaptation. It is about admitting the emotions, finding support, and eventually changing into a mindset that welcomes the potential of a life well-managed. As individuals negotiate this phase, they create the framework for the practical and emotional tools that will empower them in the continuous journey toward optimal health.

Embracing a Positive Mindset

Embracing a positive mindset following a diabetes diagnosis is a transforming activity that affects not just emotional well-being but also shapes the direction of one's health journey. The initial shock of the diagnosis generally gives way to a variety of emotions, and at this time, maintaining a positive mentality becomes a vital component of adapting to the new reality.

Positivity does not discount the problems provided by diabetes but rather reframes them as possibilities for growth and resilience. It is about knowing that a positive mindset is not the absence of obstacles but the ability to navigate them with grace and optimism. By choosing to focus on possibilities rather than constraints, individuals establish the framework for a more powerful reaction to their health conditions.

Acknowledging the adaptive potential of a positive mindset, individuals can create a sense of agency in their health journey. Rather than feeling overwhelmed by the diagnosis, a positive mentality encourages individuals to actively engage in decision-making, accept lifestyle changes, and take ownership of their well-being. It is a purposeful choice to regard the glass as half full, even in the face of obstacles.

Furthermore, a positive outlook encourages perseverance in the face of adversity. Diabetes management is a dynamic process with its share of ups and downs. Embracing an optimistic mindset enables individuals to negotiate setbacks as momentary challenges rather than insurmountable problems. This resilience becomes a useful tool in supporting long-term health goals.

Building a support system becomes a vital element of sustaining a good outlook. Surrounding oneself with understanding friends, family, and healthcare experts provides an environment that encourages optimism. Sharing triumphs, discussing obstacles, and seeking direction from this support network add to the growth of a positive and forward-thinking mindset.

In the journey towards optimal health, developing a positive mindset is not about dismissing the realities of diabetes but about redefining them. It is an intentional decision to face each day with a spirit of optimism, resilience, and a belief in the possibilities for positive change. As individuals continue to adapt and handle the intricacies of diabetes, a positive mentality becomes a guiding force, molding their response to difficulties and establishing a foundation for long-term well-being.

Chapter 2

Building Your Diabetes Support System

Establishing a comprehensive diabetes support system is a key factor in handling the obstacles that come with a diabetes diagnosis. This network, comprising family, friends, and healthcare professionals, acts as a vital pillar in the journey towards optimal health.

Within this support system, communication is key. An open and honest discussion with loved ones increases knowledge and awareness of the difficulties of diabetes. By disclosing the diagnosis and its ramifications, individuals not only obtain emotional support but also create an informed environment where everyone is aligned in supporting the necessary lifestyle changes.

Family, being an inherent element of this system, can play a significant role in giving practical aid. From meal planning to incorporating physical activity into everyday activities, involving family members in the practical aspects of diabetes care promotes a sense of unity and shared responsibility. Their engagement helps to a supportive culture that underscores the value of health-oriented choices.

Friends, too, represent a crucial component of the support system. Their empathy and support can make a huge impact on an individual's emotional well-being. Educating friends about diabetes helps debunk stereotypes and provides an environment where social activities may still be enjoyed with appropriate considerations for health.

Healthcare professionals, with their experience, become trusted allies in this support system. Regular check-ins, frank discussions about treatment plans, and requesting help on lifestyle modifications ensure that persons are well-informed and receive the required medical care. This collaborative partnership boosts the overall effectiveness of diabetes management.

Beyond personal ties, the broader diabetic community gives an extra layer of support. Engaging with support groups, both in-person and online, provides a venue for individuals to share experiences, exchange insights, and garner vital guidance from those who have traversed similar issues. These groups generate a sense of kinship, telling members that they are not alone on their path.

Developing a diabetes support system is about forging connections that transcend the confines of the illness. It is a collective effort where individuals, surrounded by understanding and encouragement, discover strength in unity. This support system, covering family, friends, and healthcare professionals, becomes a vital resource in the continual pursuit of maximum health and well-being.

The Role of Family and Friends

The role of family and friends in the area of diabetes management is vital, offering not just emotional support but also playing an active part in defining the day-to-day aspects of an individual's health journey. As a diagnosis of diabetes typically drives lifestyle alterations, the engagement and understanding of close relationships become key aspects of maintaining a supportive environment.

Family, as the fundamental nucleus of support, occupies a major role in the management of diabetes. Their comprehension of the disease can considerably influence the emotional well-being of the individual. Open communication within the family unit regarding the obstacles, nutritional demands, and lifestyle adaptations required helps create an atmosphere where everyone is aligned in supporting the individual's health goals.

Beyond emotional support, the practical engagement of family members is crucial. Involvement in food planning, support for regular physical exercise, and engagement in health-related decisions contribute to a collaborative approach. The collaborative efforts of the family not only reduce the stress on the individual but also strengthen the common commitment to overall well-being.

Friends, too, play a key role in the support system. Their empathy and encouragement contribute to the social and emotional components of diabetes care. Educating friends about the disease helps eliminate preconceptions, fostering an environment where social activities remain pleasurable and inclusive.

As individuals adapt to lifestyle changes, the support and encouragement from friends become a source of motivation. Whether it's participating in physical activities together or making informed choices during social gatherings, friends can favorably impact an individual's adherence to health-oriented behaviors.

The function of family and friends extends beyond simply companionship; it becomes an active involvement in the goal of health and well-being. The empathy, encouragement, and practical assistance afforded by these intimate relationships create a firm foundation for persons navigating the complications of diabetes. This joint effort not only enhances the quality of life for the individual but reinforces the idea that diabetes management is a shared duty within the fabric of interpersonal interactions.

Connecting with Healthcare Professionals

Connecting with healthcare specialists is a cornerstone in the entire management of diabetes, enabling an organized and informed strategy to negotiate the intricacies of the condition. The interaction between individuals and their healthcare team, often comprised of doctors, nurses, dietitians, and other professionals, creates a key partnership aimed at obtaining optimal health results.

Regular communication with healthcare providers ensures a continual and educated understanding of one's diabetes treatment plan. Routine check-ups provide an opportunity to discuss blood sugar levels, assess the effectiveness of prescribed medications, and address any growing concerns or queries. This continual communication is vital for adapting the treatment approach to the individual's particular needs.

Healthcare experts play a vital role in teaching individuals about diabetes, offering insights into the condition's subtleties, and providing advice on lifestyle adjustments. This knowledge exchange helps individuals to make informed decisions regarding diet, exercise, and other elements of everyday life, building a sense of agency in their health journey.

For those on medication, adherence to prescribed regimens is vital for good diabetes treatment. Regular check-ins with healthcare specialists allow for adjustments to drugs or dosages as needed, ensuring that the treatment plan matches the individual's growing health status. This collaborative approach contributes to the overall success of diabetes care.

In addition to medical concerns, healthcare providers offer emotional support, knowing the psychological dimensions of living with diabetes. Addressing concerns about mental well-being, coping methods, and the emotional effect of the diagnosis is a vital element of the comprehensive treatment provided by the healthcare team.

Furthermore, healthcare professionals work as champions for preventative treatment, highlighting the significance of frequent screenings and health evaluations. Monitoring for potential complications connected with diabetes, such as cardiovascular troubles or kidney problems, becomes a proactive tool in maintaining long-term health.

Connecting with healthcare providers fosters a dynamic collaboration that extends beyond the clinical setting. It is a cooperation focused on open communication, mutual respect, and a shared commitment to achieving and sustaining optimal health. This partnership becomes a guiding force, giving the necessary tools, education, and support for individuals to traverse the difficult landscape of diabetes control.

Exploring Diabetes Communities

Exploring diabetes communities serves as a vital component of the broader strategy for treating this chronic condition, allowing patients a sense of connection, shared experiences, and a plethora of helpful information. These communities, whether in-person or online, establish a friendly environment where persons with diabetes, their families, and caregivers may join together to share information and encouragement.

Participating in diabetic communities offers a unique opportunity for individuals to connect with others who are facing similar issues. Sharing personal experiences, including achievements and challenges, promotes a sense of solidarity and understanding. This sense of community can be particularly effective in fighting feelings of isolation that patients with chronic diseases may experience.

One of the primary advantages of diabetes groups is the exchange of practical information and tips for managing daily life. From navigating food choices to discussing effective exercise regimens, community members give practical expertise that goes beyond typical medical counsel. This peer-to-peer support can be a beneficial supplement to conventional healthcare guidance.

Online platforms, forums, and social media groups dedicated to diabetes give accessible areas for individuals to seek help and share their adventures. The convenience of connecting with a varied range of persons from various backgrounds and experiences expands the breadth of information available, allowing individuals to personalize their approach to diabetes care based on a more comprehensive understanding.

Within these networks, individuals typically find a safe area to explore the emotional elements of living with diabetes. Whether sharing personal successes or discussing the obstacles of sustaining mental well-being, the empathy and compassion within these groups offer an environment where individuals may openly express their thoughts and feelings.

Moreover, diabetic communities serve as a resource hub for remaining informed about the newest breakthroughs in diabetes research, treatment options, and lifestyle suggestions. This collective knowledge helps individuals to make informed decisions about their health and to stay current on advances that may affect their diabetes care.

Exploring diabetes communities gives a gateway to a wealth of support, education, and shared experiences. The relationships made within these groups contribute not just to the practical aspects of diabetes care but also to the emotional well-being of those navigating the complexity of life with diabetes.

Chapter 3

Nutrition for Diabetes Control

Nutrition stands as a cornerstone in the proper management of diabetes, playing a key role in managing blood sugar levels and maintaining general well-being. Understanding the influence of dietary choices on glucose levels is vital for those with diabetes, and adopting a strategic approach to nutrition becomes a key element of their daily routine.

Carbohydrates, being a key source of energy, considerably influence blood sugar levels. Managing the quantity and quality of carbs is critical for diabetic control. Emphasizing complex carbs having a lower glycemic index, such as whole grains, vegetables, and legumes, assists in maintaining more stable blood sugar levels compared to simple carbohydrates found in processed foods.

The distribution of carbs throughout the day also has a role in glycemic management. Spreading carbohydrate intake throughout meals can minimize rapid rises in blood sugar levels. Additionally, mixing carbohydrates with protein and healthy fats might further slowdown the absorption of glucose, helping to better blood sugar regulation.

Portion control is a crucial component in diabetes nutrition. Maintaining appropriate portion sizes helps regulate calorie intake and prevents overconsumption, supporting weight management — a vital component of diabetes care. Monitoring portion sizes, especially of high-calorie foods, adds to both blood sugar control and overall health.

Beyond carbohydrates, paying attention to the quality of fats is vital. Choosing heart-healthy fats, such as those found in avocados, almonds, and olive oil, adds to cardiovascular health, which is particularly essential for those with diabetes who may be at a higher risk of heart-related issues.

Protein intake, sourced from lean meats, poultry, fish, and plant-based choices, is another key part of the diabetes diet. Protein not only promotes muscular health but also aids in managing appetite and encouraging fullness, adding to weight management goals.

The value of fiber cannot be emphasized in diabetes-friendly eating. High-fiber meals, including fruits, vegetables, and whole grains, not only supply critical nutrients but also aid in better blood sugar regulation by slowing down the digestion and absorption of carbs.

Nutrition for diabetes control is a complex approach that incorporates intelligent decisions in carbohydrate, lipid, and protein intake, as well as an emphasis on portion control and dietary fiber. By implementing these ideas into daily life, individuals with diabetes can proactively manage their condition and enhance overall health and well-being.

Mastering Diabetes-Friendly Eating

Mastering diabetes-friendly eating is a dynamic and inspiring path that entails adopting a holistic approach to nutrition, taking into account the special needs of individuals living with diabetes. This mastery is not about restricting diets but rather about making informed and sustainable decisions that contribute to optimal blood sugar control and general well-being.

At the heart of learning a diabetes-friendly diet is understanding the glycemic impact of different foods. The glycemic index (GI) is a handy tool for analyzing how rapidly a particular diet elevates blood sugar levels. Incorporating low-GI foods, such as whole grains, non-starchy vegetables, and legumes, into the diet encourages a steady and regulated release of glucose, helping to minimize rapid surges.

Balancing macronutrients — carbohydrates, proteins, and fats – becomes a vital component of understanding a diabetes-friendly diet. While carbohydrates are carefully handled, it's crucial not to forget the importance of proteins and fats. Including lean protein sources, such as poultry, fish, and tofu, and incorporating healthy fats from sources like avocados and almonds, adds diversity and nutritional value to meals while boosting overall health.

Portion control remains a vital discipline in mastering diabetes-friendly eating. Being careful of serving sizes helps limit calorie intake, helping with weight management and, ultimately, improved blood sugar control. This consideration of portion sizes extends to snacks, ensuring that they correspond with overall nutritional goals and do not upset the delicate balance of blood sugar levels.

Strategic meal planning is a critical component of learning diabetes-friendly eating. Structuring meals with a combination of carbohydrates, proteins, and fats, and spacing them throughout the day, helps maintain stable blood sugar levels. This method reduces excessive changes in glucose, promoting greater control over diabetes.

Diversifying food choices within the framework of diabetes-friendly eating adds richness to the diet. Experimenting with a range of fruits, vegetables, whole grains, and lean proteins not only boosts nutritional intake but also makes the experience of healthy eating more enjoyable and sustainable over the long run.

Furthermore, staying hydrated is often ignored yet is crucial to a diabetes-friendly diet. Opting for water and other low-calorie, sugar-free beverages boosts general health and aids in keeping optimal hydration levels.

Mastering a diabetes-friendly diet includes acquiring a comprehensive grasp of the impact of different foods on blood sugar levels. It is a journey of balance, diversity, and informed choices that enable individuals to take care of their health while enjoying a diversified and enjoyable diet.

Understanding Glycemic Index

Understanding the Glycemic Index (GI) is a vital feature of regulating blood sugar levels and making informed food decisions, particularly for persons with diabetes. The Glycemic Index is a ranking system that categorizes foods based on how rapidly they cause blood sugar to rise after eating. This numerical scale, often ranging from 0 to 100, classifies foods as low, medium, or high on the glycemic index.

Low-GI foods, with a score below 55, are those that promote a gradual and regulated increase in blood sugar levels. Examples of low-GI foods comprise of non-starchy vegetables, legumes, and whole grains. Incorporating these foods into the diet helps maintain stable blood sugar levels and delivers a sustained supply of energy.

Medium-GI meals, with a score between 56 and 69, generate a mild increase in blood sugar levels. Foods like whole-wheat products and select fruits fall into this group. While these foods can be part of a balanced diet, it's crucial to take them in moderation and be conscious of their impact on blood sugar.

High-GI meals, with a score of 70 or above, produce a quick surge in blood sugar levels. Examples include sugary cereals, white bread, and certain processed foods. Limiting the intake of high-GI foods is critical for patients with diabetes to minimize rapid rises and reductions in blood sugar, supporting better overall control.

Understanding the Glycemic Index is not about eliminating entire food groups but rather making strategic decisions within them. Combining low-GI meals with sources of lean protein and healthy fats can further regulate the overall influence on blood sugar levels, contributing to a more balanced and diabetes-friendly diet.

It's vital to note that the Glycemic Index is not a single aspect to consider. The Glycemic Load (GL), which takes into consideration both the quality and quantity of carbs in a meal, gives a more comprehensive assessment of a food's impact on blood sugar.

Understanding the Glycemic Index helps individuals to make aware and informed judgments regarding their dietary choices. By including low and moderate-GI foods in their meals, individuals with diabetes can encourage better blood sugar management and establish the groundwork for a balanced and sustainable approach to nutrition.

Crafting Balanced Meals

Crafting balanced meals is an art that goes beyond addressing hunger needs; it is a systematic approach to nutrition that plays a critical role in sustaining overall health, particularly for persons with diabetes. Balancing macronutrients – carbohydrates, proteins, and fats – within a meal is crucial in establishing stable blood sugar levels and sustaining long-term well-being.

The foundation of a balanced meal frequently starts with choosing a variety of colorful and nutrient-rich veggies. These non-starchy veggies give critical vitamins, minerals, and fiber while providing a pleasant and tasty component to the plate. Their low-calorie content makes them an ideal choice for people working on weight management.

Incorporating lean protein sources is a critical feature of making balanced meals. Protein not only maintains muscle function but also plays a critical role in satiety, helping individuals feel full and satisfied after a meal. Options such as poultry, fish, tofu, lentils, and low-fat dairy products give numerous and nutritious choices for protein intake.

Careful assessment of carbohydrate choices is crucial, especially for persons with diabetes. Opting for complex carbs with a lower Glycemic Index, such as whole grains, quinoa, and sweet potatoes, encourages a slow release of glucose into the bloodstream, reducing abrupt rises in blood sugar levels.

Including healthy fats in the form of avocados, nuts, seeds, and olive oil offers vital fatty acids and adds a delicious dimension to meals. These fats add to a feeling of fullness and aid in the absorption of fat-soluble vitamins.

Portion control is a guiding principle in constructing balanced meals, ensuring that calorie intake fits with individual nutritional goals. Paying attention to portion sizes helps regulate energy consumption, helping both blood sugar regulation and weight management.

The timing of meals is another issue in the building of balanced meals. Spreading food consumption across the day, with frequent meals and snacks, helps maintain stable blood sugar levels and minimizes excessive variations.

Crafting balanced meals is about synergy and deliberate decisions. It entails selecting a combination of nutrient-dense foods that contribute to overall health while considering the special needs of those with diabetes. By approaching meal planning with a strategic attitude, individuals can proactively manage their blood sugar levels and build a sustainable and enjoyable approach to nutrition.

Portion Control Strategies

Portion management stands as a vital feature of keeping a healthy and balanced diet, and for persons managing diabetes, it becomes an extremely crucial component in regulating blood sugar levels. Adopting successful portion management tactics is not about deprivation but rather about making thoughtful decisions that improve overall well-being.

One of the primary methods in portion management is to be conscious of serving sizes. Familiarizing oneself with normal serving sizes, as recommended by dietary standards, provides a solid reference point for assessing the amount of food consumed. This awareness helps minimize unintended overeating and adds to a more accurate assessment of calorie intake.

Another good method is to use smaller dishes and bowls. The visual sense of a full plate can alter the brain's perception of satiety. By opting for smaller dishware, individuals are more likely to feel satisfied with suitably sized meals, minimizing the urge to overeat.

Taking the time to taste each bite and eat slowly is a conscious approach to portion control. This method permits the body's natural signals of fullness to catch up with the pace of eating, fostering a greater awareness of when to stop. Engaging in conversation during meals and laying down utensils between bites are practical strategies to encourage a slower eating speed.

Measuring and measuring food amounts, especially when starting on a portion control journey, provides an accurate way to comprehend portion proportions. Using measuring cups or a food scale for a period can help individuals develop an instinctive feel of portion proportions, making it easier to eyeball meals in the future.

Choosing nutrient-dense foods is an approach that naturally fits with portion control. Nutrient-dense foods, such as fruits, vegetables, lean proteins, and whole grains, supply important vitamins and minerals without excessive calories. Prioritizing these items allows folks to enjoy greater servings while still keeping a balanced diet.

The discipline of mindful eating entails paying attention to hunger and fullness indicators. Understanding the body's signals and eating in reaction to hunger, rather than external cues, creates a healthier relationship with food. It also encourages individuals to quit eating when comfortably content, eliminating excessive overconsumption.

Portion control tactics are practical tools that empower individuals to make informed choices regarding the quantity of food they consume. By integrating these practices into daily life, individuals can achieve better blood sugar control, promote weight management, and build a sustained approach to healthy eating.

Chapter 4

Meal Planning and Preparation

Meal planning and preparation serve as pillars in the foundation of a well-rounded and health-conscious approach to nutrition. For individuals managing diabetes, these activities become even more vital, providing an organized strategy to make thoughtful choices and maintain stable blood sugar levels.

Central to efficient meal planning is the emphasis on diversity. Planning meals that incorporate a broader variety of food categories ensures that individuals receive a broad spectrum of critical nutrients. This diversity not only benefits general health but also provides a richness of flavors and textures to the dining experience, making meals more enjoyable.

Setting up devoted time for meal planning allows individuals to examine their dietary objectives, tastes, and nutritional requirements. It provides an opportunity to mindfully select dishes, guaranteeing a balance of carbohydrates, proteins, and fats. Additionally, preparing ahead allows for a more systematic approach to portion control and helps avoid impulsive, less health-conscious eating choices.

A vital part of good meal planning is the incorporation of nutrient-dense meals. Fruits, vegetables, nutritious grains, and lean proteins constitute the backbone of a well-balanced diet plan. These meals not only supply critical vitamins and minerals but also help to prolonged energy release, enabling better blood sugar regulation throughout the day.

In the area of diabetes control, mindful carbohydrate counting is often part of the meal planning process. Being mindful of the carbohydrate content in foods and dividing them equally between meals helps prevent rapid rises in blood sugar levels. This strategic approach to carbohydrate intake aligns with the broader goal of keeping a constant glucose profile.

Meal preparation is the practical execution of the meal planning strategy. This involves chores such as chopping vegetables, marinating proteins, and pre-portioning items. Setting aside time for meal preparation not only streamlines the cooking process but also encourages healthier choices by having readily available, well-prepared options.

Incorporating batch cooking into the meal preparation routine is a time-saving method. Cooking bigger portions of certain recipes allows for leftovers that can be used for following meals. This technique not only lowers the time spent in the kitchen but also provides a continuous supply of healthful and balanced alternatives throughout the week.

Meal planning and preparation are active instruments in the arsenal of diabetes control. They encourage individuals to take charge of their food choices, creating a proactive and intentional attitude to nutrition. By integrating these techniques into their routine, individuals can navigate the complications of diabetes with a focus on health, diversity, and the delight of savoring tasty, well-thought-out meals.

Creating Weekly Meal Plans

Creating weekly meal planning is a deliberate and empowering technique that develops both discipline and flexibility in one's approach to nutrition. For individuals managing diabetes, this planning becomes a vital tool in achieving optimal blood sugar management and maintaining a balanced diet.

The cornerstone of a weekly meal plan frequently starts with an assessment of dietary goals and nutritional needs. This includes concerns about calorie consumption, macronutrient distribution, and particular tastes. Understanding these factors gives a blueprint for developing meals that correspond with both health objectives and personal interests.

Variety is an important aspect of establishing weekly food plans. Diversifying meal choices ensures a wide array of nutrients and eliminates dietary monotony. Planning meals with a mix of different proteins, whole grains, fruits, and vegetables not only increases nutritional intake but also enriches the whole dining experience.

Mindful carbohydrate counting is a key component in the weekly meal planning process for those with diabetes. Distributing carbohydrates evenly across meals helps manage blood sugar levels. By selectively incorporating high-fiber, low-GI meals, the meal plan can contribute to continuous energy release throughout the day.

Considering the practicalities of daily life is key to designing realistic and feasible weekly meal plans. This requires factoring in time limits, potential leftovers, and the balance between home-cooked and convenience options. A pragmatic approach to planning ensures that the food plan matches with the individual's lifestyle.

Batch cooking emerges as a beneficial method in the context of weekly meal plans. Preparing larger portions of certain recipes provides for leftovers that can be utilized for later meals. This not only speeds the cooking process but also provides a steady supply of well-prepared, diabetes-friendly meals throughout the week.

Incorporating seasonal and local products into the weekly meal plan adds both freshness and nutritional value to meals. This strategy not only supports local agriculture but also provides an opportunity to taste a range of fruits and vegetables at their best flavor and nutritious content.

Flexibility within the structure of the weekly meal plan is crucial. While planning gives a roadmap, being open to alterations based on daily conditions or unforeseen events allows for a practical and sustainable strategy. Flexibility also increases adaptation, making it simpler to sustain good eating habits in the long run.

Creating weekly meal planning is a dynamic and proactive method that encourages individuals to take control of their nutritional choices. By incorporating variety, attentive carbohydrate counting, and practical considerations, individuals can navigate the week with a focus on both health and fun, contributing to the greater objective of optimal diabetes management.

Smart Grocery Shopping for Diabetes

Smart grocery shopping for diabetes is a proactive and strategic method that helps consumers make informed decisions that correspond with their health goals. Navigating the aisles with mindfulness, knowledge, and a focus on nutrient-dense products is crucial to maintaining overall well-being, particularly for those managing diabetes.

One of the core concepts of sensible food shopping is to plan ahead. Before traveling to the market, taking the time to make a precise shopping list based on a weekly meal plan helps consumers get what they need and prevents impulsive selections. This method not only streamlines the shopping process but also helps to a more planned and health-conscious approach to meals.

Prioritizing fresh produce is a cornerstone of wise grocery shopping for diabetes. Fruits and vegetables, rich in vitamins, minerals, and fiber, provide the cornerstone of a balanced diet. Opting for a variety of colors and varieties ensures a wide spectrum of nutrients, boosting general health and well-being. Additionally, picking seasonal and local produce generally boosts both flavor and nutritional content.

Navigating the carbohydrate aisle with mindfulness is vital for persons managing diabetes. Selecting whole grains, such as quinoa, brown rice, and whole wheat products, gives a healthier option to refined grains. Checking food labels for added sugars and opting for goods with high fiber content aids improved blood sugar control.

The protein department offers an opportunity to make lean and healthful choices. Incorporating sources such as lean poultry, fish, tofu, and lentils gives needed amino acids without excessive saturated fats. For those who consume meat, choosing lean cuts and eliminating visible fat help heart health, an important concern for those with diabetes.

Reading food labels becomes a skill in savvy grocery shopping. Checking nutritional information for total carbohydrates, fiber levels, and portion sizes assists in making informed choices. Being careful of hidden sugars, sodium, and bad fats allows individuals to select goods that match with their dietary needs and health objectives.

The perimeter of the grocery store frequently holds fresh produce, dairy, and lean proteins. While visiting the interior aisles is vital, focusing on the outside edges supports a diet rich in whole and less processed foods. This strategy emphasizes a nutrient-dense and balanced selection of items for a well-rounded meal plan.

Smart grocery shopping for diabetes needs a combination of planning, awareness, and conscious choices. By prioritizing fresh, complete foods and being conscious of nutritional information, consumers can change their grocery shopping experience into a proactive step towards efficient diabetes control and general health

Cooking Techniques for Diabetes-Friendly Meals

Mastering cooking techniques is a useful tool for those managing diabetes, allowing them to prepare delicious and diabetes-friendly meals while retaining control over crucial nutritional ingredients. A number of cooking methods can be applied to enhance flavors, conserve nutrients, and increase overall health.

Grilling is a popular technique that provides a characteristic Smokey flavor to dishes without the need for excessive fats. Lean foods like chicken, fish, and vegetables may be grilled to perfection, resulting in delightful and health-conscious selections. It's crucial to marinade things with tasty, low-sugar sauces to provide depth without violating nutritional goals.

Baking and roasting are diverse processes that allow an opportunity to accentuate natural flavors. By adding herbs, spices, and a small amount of heart-healthy oils, folks can make foods with pleasant textures and scents. These approaches are particularly ideal for vegetables, lean meats, and whole grains, contributing to a well-balanced and diabetes-friendly dinner.

Sautéing enables rapid and tasty cooking with tiny amounts of oil. It's a fantastic approach for veggies, lean proteins, and even certain grains. Choosing heart-healthy oils like olive oil boosts the nutritional profile of the dish, supplying vital fatty acids without excessive saturated fats.

Steaming is a mild cooking method that preserves the natural colors and nutrients of vegetables, making it a great technique for individuals controlling diabetes. From broccoli to asparagus, steaming keeps the crispness of food while ensuring they are cooked to perfection. It's a simple yet efficient way to generate a nutrient-rich supper.

Poaching includes gradually cooking items in a delicious liquid, commonly water or broth. This technique is great for cooking proteins like fish or chicken without extra lipids. Poached products can be coupled with herbs and spices to boost the taste while sticking to diabetes-friendly dietary requirements.

Stir-frying provides for a speedy and lively cooking procedure, making it a good choice for busy folks managing diabetes. Using a small amount of oil and integrating an array of bright veggies, lean proteins, and whole grains provides a visually pleasing and nutritionally sound dish.

Slow cooking is a practical method that requires less hands-on time. By blending lean proteins, vegetables, and nutritious grains in a slow cooker, folks can make tender and tasty meals. This strategy is useful for people wishing to maintain control over their food without continual observation.

Incorporating these cooking techniques into one's culinary repertoire not only enhances the enjoyment of meals but also promotes diabetes management goals. By focusing on fresh, whole foods and experimenting with various approaches, individuals can build a broad and enjoyable array of diabetes-friendly dishes that highlight both taste and nutritional value.

Chapter 5

Active Living for Diabetes Wellness

Active living is an essential element of diabetes wellness, giving a plethora of physical and emotional health advantages for persons managing diabetes. Engaging in regular physical activity is not only vital for blood sugar control but also contributes to overall well-being and illness management.

Aerobic workouts, such as brisk walking, cycling, or swimming, have a crucial role in diabetes control. These exercises assist enhance insulin sensitivity, allowing cells to effectively utilize glucose. Regular aerobic exercise also benefits in weight management, reducing the risk of insulin resistance and cardiovascular issues associated with diabetes.

Strength training is another vital component of an active lifestyle for those with diabetes. Building muscular mass not only boosts metabolism but also leads to better blood sugar management. Resistance exercises, such as weightlifting or bodyweight workouts, assist individuals to maintain healthy body composition and support overall metabolic health.

Flexibility and balanced activities are vital for diabetes well-being, especially as people age. Activities like yoga or tai chi not only develop flexibility and balance but also promote stress reduction. Stress management is critical for those with diabetes since stress can affect blood sugar levels and general health.

Incorporating physical activity into daily life is crucial for maintaining diabetes health. Simple lifestyle modifications, such as taking the stairs, walking instead of driving short distances, or implementing short bursts of activity throughout the day, contribute to total activity levels. These simple alterations can have a substantial influence on blood sugar control and long-term health.

Engaging in activities that bring joy and contentment is crucial for keeping an active lifestyle. Whether it's dancing, gardening, or participating in recreational sports, choosing activities that folks actually like creates a sustainable and joyful attitude to physical activity. This not only contributes to diabetes management but also promotes general quality of life.

Regular monitoring of blood sugar levels before and after physical activity is critical for those with diabetes. This enables modifications in medication, food intake, or activity levels to maintain optimal blood sugar management during and after exercise. Consulting with healthcare professionals ensures a targeted approach that corresponds with individual health goals.

Active living is a crucial part of diabetes wellness. By adding a variety of physical activities into everyday life, individuals can increase their general health, support blood sugar control, and lower the risk of diabetes-related problems. The route toward diabetes wellness is paved with the simple yet revolutionary act of embracing an active and rewarding lifestyle.

Exercise Essentials for Diabetes Management

Exercise stands as a cornerstone in the effective management of diabetes, giving a range of advantages that transcend physical fitness. Understanding the principles of exercise for diabetes management helps individuals make informed decisions that favorably improve blood sugar control and general health.

Aerobic exercise, commonly known as cardiovascular exercise, is crucial for patients with diabetes. Activities like brisk walking, cycling, swimming, or dancing boost the heart rate and promote circulation. Regular aerobic exercise raises insulin sensitivity, allowing cells to effectively utilize glucose. This contributes to improved blood sugar control and minimizes the risk of cardiovascular problems linked to diabetes.

Strength training is a vital component of diabetes management. Building and maintaining muscular mass not only enhances metabolism but also aids in glucose usage. Resistance exercises, such as weightlifting or bodyweight workouts, have a key role in reducing insulin resistance and boosting overall metabolic health. Individuals should strive for at least two sessions of strength training per week.

Flexibility exercises are often disregarded, yet they are vital for diabetes wellness. Engaging in activities that develop flexibility, such as yoga or stretching regimens, promotes joint mobility and minimizes the chance of accidents. These activities also assist in stress reduction, an important aspect of diabetes control, as stress can alter blood sugar levels.

Balancing exercises, such as tai chi or specific yoga positions, promote stability and minimize the risk of falls, which is particularly crucial for those with diabetes who may develop neuropathy or other issues affecting balance. Incorporating balance exercises into a regimen helps preserve general physical function and minimizes the chance of injuries.

Individualization is crucial when establishing an exercise plan for diabetes treatment. Considering personal preferences, fitness levels, and any underlying health conditions enables a tailored approach that individuals are more likely to sustain. It's vital to work with healthcare professionals, including physicians and experienced fitness trainers, to design a safe and successful exercise regimen.

Monitoring blood sugar levels before, during, and after exercise is critical. This helps patients understand how different activities influence their blood sugar and allows for adjustments in medication, food consumption, or exercise intensity accordingly. Consistent monitoring provides vital insights into the individual's response to exercise, supporting better diabetes treatment.

Integrating physical activity into daily life is equally vital. Simple lifestyle modifications, such as taking the stairs, walking instead of driving short distances, or implementing short bursts of activity throughout the day, contribute to total activity levels. These minor alterations, when persistent, can greatly improve blood sugar control.

Exercise is a key tool in the diabetes management repertoire. By adopting a combination of aerobic, strength, flexibility, and balancing activities, individuals can boost their general health, support blood sugar control, and lower the risk of diabetes-related problems. The elements of exercise for diabetes control lie in a personalized and holistic approach that matches individual health objectives and preferences.

Developing a Personalized Exercise Plan

Creating a personalized fitness plan is a vital step in optimizing diabetes management and general well-being. This individualized approach ensures that individuals may include physical exercise into their lives in a way that matches their unique requirements, preferences, and health goals.

1. Assessing Current Fitness Levels: The first step in establishing a personalized workout plan is to measure current fitness levels. This requires considering aspects such as cardiovascular fitness, strength, flexibility, and overall health. A full examination gives a baseline from which to create reasonable and achievable goals.

2. Establishing Clear Goals: Clearly defined goals serve as a guide for the fitness strategy. Whether the focus is on improving cardiovascular health, increasing strength, enhancing flexibility, or attaining weight management, having defined and quantifiable goals provides direction and incentive.

3. Choosing Enjoyable Activities: Incorporating activities that individuals actually love boosts the likelihood of commitment to the fitness plan. Whether it's walking, cycling, swimming, dancing, or engaging in sports, selecting activities that provide joy ensures a more sustainable and enjoyable approach to physical activity.

4. Balancing Aerobic, Strength, and Flexibility Exercises:

A well-rounded workout routine contains a combination of aerobic, strength, and flexibility exercises. Aerobic activities increase cardiovascular health, strength training supports muscle mass and metabolism, and flexibility exercises promote joint health. Balancing these components helps with overall fitness.

5. Gradual Progression: Gradual progression is crucial, especially for individuals beginning to fitness or returning after a time of inactivity. Starting with moderate durations and intensities helps prevent injuries and allows the body to adjust progressively. Over time, the training routine can be changed to match increased fitness levels.

6. Considering Time Limits: Recognizing time limits and integrating physical exercise into daily life is vital for long-term commitment. Developing a strategy that fits into one's schedule, whether through quick bursts of activity, planned workouts, or a combination of both, offers a more realistic and sustainable approach.

7. Monitoring Blood Sugar Levels: Regular monitoring of blood sugar levels before, during, and after exercise is critical for those with diabetes. This approach helps understand how different activities affect blood sugar and enables for modifications in medication, dietary consumption, or exercise intensity to maintain optimal control.

8. Seeking Professional Guidance: Consulting with healthcare specialists, including physicians and qualified fitness trainers, provides vital insights and ensures that the activity plan matches individual health issues. Professional guidance helps address unique health concerns, adapting the approach for the best safety and effectiveness.

9. Incorporating Rest and Recovery: Building rest and recovery into the training regimen is vital for reducing burnout and increasing general well-being. Adequate rest allows the body to recover and adapt to the demands of physical activity, lowering the risk of weariness or overuse problems.

Developing a tailored fitness plan is a dynamic and individualized process. By measuring existing fitness levels, defining clear goals, choosing pleasant activities, and balancing different types of workouts, individuals can design a plan that not only improves diabetes control but also fosters a lifelong commitment to a healthy and active lifestyle.

Overcoming Barriers to Physical Activity

Embarking on the journey towards regular physical activity might be accompanied by many challenges, but conquering these barriers is vital for prolonged health and well-being. Understanding and resolving these challenges allows individuals to develop a more accessible path to incorporate exercise into their daily lives.

1. Lack of Time: A major barrier to physical activity is a perceived lack of time in our fast-paced lives. However, knowing that physical activity doesn't necessarily require extended time can be a game-changer. Short, concentrated workouts or integrating movement into regular routines, such as using the stairs or walking during breaks, might successfully address this difficulty.

2. Motivational Hurdles: Maintaining motivation can be a struggle, especially when faced with the pressures of daily life. Establishing clear and realistic goals, recognizing little accomplishments, and choosing hobbies that bring joy are key to keeping motivated. Incorporating social factors, such as exercising with a friend or taking group programs, can provide further inspiration.

3. Physical limits or Health Concerns: Individuals with physical limits or health concerns may see exercise as overwhelming. However, engaging with healthcare specialists to select safe and suitable activities is crucial. Tailoring a workout regimen to fit unique health factors ensures a more inclusive and individualized approach.

4. Lack of Access to Facilities: Limited access to exercise facilities might represent a barrier, particularly in specific geographical locations. However, physical exercise doesn't always necessitate a gym membership. Outdoor activities, home workouts, or utilizing community areas can give accessible alternatives. Making the most of available resources encourages adaptation.

5. Weather circumstances: Weather circumstances might affect outdoor exercise plans, potentially preventing folks from keeping active. However, having a choice of indoor workout options or adapting outside activities to varied weather conditions, such as walking indoors or doing yoga at home, allows for flexibility and sustained involvement.

6. Family or job duties: Balancing family or job duties may make finding time for exercise seem tough. Incorporating physical activity into family routines, incorporating loved ones in activities, or emphasizing short, targeted workouts throughout hectic days might assist overcome this obstacle. Recognizing the benefits of self-care contributes to a more holistic approach to health.

7. Lack of enthusiasm or Variety: A lack of enthusiasm in traditional exercises can limit commitment. Finding activities that correspond with personal interests or trying a range of routines might make the experience more enjoyable. Whether it's dancing, hiking, or trying new sports, recognizing what offers joy is crucial in developing a lasting commitment to physical activity.

8. Financial limits: Financial limits may limit access to some fitness options. However, several cost-effective or free alternatives excesses, from walking and running to employing Internet workout resources. Exploring cheap solutions ensures that financial considerations don't become an impediment to keeping an active lifestyle.

9. Fear of Judgment: Fear of judgment, especially for individuals new to exercise or with specific body image concerns, can be a substantial barrier. Recognizing that everyone has distinct fitness paths and that there is no one-size-fits-all method can help individuals overcome self-consciousness. Creating a supportive atmosphere, whether personally or as a group, develops inclusion.

Overcoming impediments to physical activity involves a combination of practical answers and a mental adjustment. By understanding unique restrictions, finding innovative solutions, and highlighting the joy and inclusion of physical activity, individuals can pave the path for a lasting and happy commitment to regular exercise

Chapter 6

Stress Reduction and Sleep Optimization

When it comes to the hectic symphony that is modern life, stress frequently takes the spotlight, playing a discordant melody that reverberates throughout our brains and bodies. Amidst the cacophony, the yearning for peace becomes important. Imagine the skillful conductor of a lovely song that reverberates with feelings of calm and tranquility as the stress reduction specialist.

The Prelude: Stress Reduction Symphony

Imagine a garden drenched in the soothing hues of sunset, where worry evaporates like morning dew. In this context, the instrumentalists are awareness and meditation, which together create a tapestry of tranquility. Every note in the orchestra is invited to resonate with the beat of the current moment by the conductor, who guides the orchestra through the gentle cadence of deep breathing.

Yoga, which involves gently stretching and untangling knots of stress, is represented by the strings in this symphony musical composition. The woodwinds reverberate the calming sounds of nature, which have the effect of transferring the mind to peaceful places. The rhythm of the percussion, which is subtle and rhythmic, is a reflection of the heartbeat of individuals who find comfort in the act of simply being.

With laughter, the unexpected virtuoso, whose lightness dispels the shadows of stress, develops into a crescendo. The music is characterized by the whimsical soloist of laughter, which dances throughout the piece to remind us that joy is a remedy for the burdens that are associated with daily life.

The Intermezzo: The Sleep Optimization Lullaby with Interlude

As the sun sets on the stress reduction symphony, the moon rises to expose the lullaby of sleep optimization. The conductor shifts, taking us through the nighttime dances, where regeneration emerges.

The overture begins with a darkening of lights, prompting the body to release the conductor's wand, melatonin. The quiet hum of a sleep-friendly environment harmonizes with the murmur of a nightly routine, establishing a spell of peace.

In this nocturne, the brass part depicts the comfort of a supportive mattress, offering the foundation for a quiet night.

The strings reverberate with the silkiness of sleepwear, a tactile sonnet that cradles the body in a cocoon of rest.

The nocturnal rhapsody takes an ethereal turn with the heavenly dance of dreams as the mind pirouettes through worlds of imagination and subconscious wanderings. Each sleep cycle, a movement in the symphony, contributes to the opus of regeneration.

Finale: A Harmonious Dawn

As the night's symphony closes, the first rays of dawn herald a new day. The maestro of stress reduction and sleep improvement, having delivered a night of restorative music, steps back. The beautiful echoes linger, guiding us into a day where tension finds no solos and sleep is an encore of vigor.

In this crescendo of well-being, the dance between stress reduction and sleep optimization intertwines, creating a song that resonates with the essence of a joyful existence. The symphony continues, a continual melody to the rhythm of a life well lived.

Stress's Impact on Diabetes

In the complicated symphony of diabetes care, stress emerges as a strong conductor, brandishing a baton that alters the rhythm of blood sugar levels. Consider this: the stage is set, the lights are muted, and stress takes center stage, orchestrating a composition that plays a key role in the diabetes tale.

The stress prelude opens with an ominous beat, prompting the release of stress hormones that flow through the body. As the anxiety-laden song unfolds, it causes a cascade effect, elevating blood sugar levels. It's a theatrical overture where the body, in response to stress, prepares for a fight-or-flight performance, typically triggering glucose surges.

The brass section vibrates with a heightened heartbeat, a tactile representation of stress's influence. The percussion follows suit, expressing the tension that tightens the muscles, leaving the body in a state of alertness. The woodwinds replicate the short, shallow breaths, a reflection of the respiratory alterations generated by stress, further altering glucose levels.

In this complicated symphony, the strings section embodies the subtle dance between stress and insulin resistance. As stress takes center stage, insulin's function is weakened, leaving glucose without a companion for its beautiful dance into the cells. The result: increased blood sugar, a solitary act that breaks the equilibrium of diabetes care.

As the Stress Symphony progresses, the audience watches the psychological motions, where stress adds to emotional eating—a subplot in the diabetic play. The stage of emotional eating is set, and stress plays the primary role, prompting individuals to seek solace in comfort foods, frequently heavy in carbohydrates. It's a captivating duet between stress and poor food choices.

The Crescendo of Cortisol, the stress hormone, steals the limelight. This hormone, analogous to a loud crescendo, not only boosts blood sugar levels but also urges the liver to release stored glucose. It's a crescendo that resonates through the metabolic corridors, disturbing the delicate balance essential for successful diabetic treatment.

As the closing notes of the Stress Symphony linger, it becomes obvious that stress is not only an accidental character but a crucial one influencing the narrative of diabetes. Understanding this complex composition helps individuals become conductors of their diabetes care, introducing counter-melodies of stress reduction and resilience.

In the big theatre of diabetes care, seeing stress as a prominent player promotes a sophisticated approach. By understanding the impact of stress, individuals can fine-tune their techniques, introducing harmonies that offset the disruptive notes. The goal is to change the Stress Symphony into a mellifluous arrangement where diabetes management takes center stage and stress plays a supporting role in the background.

Relaxation Techniques

Imagine a quiet oasis, a place where the stormy waves of stress dissolve, and tranquility takes center stage. In the arena of stress management, relaxation techniques emerge as virtuoso artists, each offering a distinctive melody to the symphony of peace.

Let's begin with the calm hum of Deep Breathing, a melody that resonates through the ages. Inhale, exhale — a rhythmic dance that synchronizes with the ebb and flow of life's demands. The diaphragm, the conductor of this calming sonnet, orchestrates a cadence that signals the nervous system to change from fight-or-flight to a state of tranquil slumber.

Picture the smooth resonance of a Guided Imagery Symphony, when the mind goes on a visual voyage to serene settings. A meandering river, sun-kissed meadows, or a starlit sky — each scene a brushstroke in the canvas of the mind. Guided imagery helps individuals build their mental retreat, a sanctuary where stress is an unwelcome guest.

Now, let the waves of stress be carried away by the Progressive Muscle Relaxation Ballet. In this choreographed sequence, muscles become the dancers, delicately releasing tension with each thoughtful movement. It's a dance of mindfulness, where the body, attuned to the beat of relaxation, unveils a performance that leaves stress in the wings.

The Mindfulness Meditation Waltz takes center stage, a dance of the present that transcends the cacophony of thoughts. In this waltz, the mind becomes sensitive to the present moment, with the dancers moving in sync with the breath. Mindfulness meditation is a timeless choreography that uncovers the elegance of being present.

Feel the resonating vibrations of the Nature Sounds Symphony, a song where the rustling leaves, babbling brooks, and singing birds build a tapestry of auditory serenity. This symphony of nature provides an audio escape, taking individuals to the peacefulness of natural settings, a harmonious reprieve from the metropolitan cacophony.

The soft plucking of strings opens the Autogenic Relaxation Sonata, a composition where individuals produce a sense of warmth and heaviness in various places of the body. It's a self-directed tune, a musical score written by the individual, inviting a sense of serenity and equilibrium.

As the relaxation techniques perform their harmonic compositions, it's vital to acknowledge the Laughter Intermezzo — a spontaneous and uninhibited burst of joy.

Laughter, the quirky soloist, requires no elaborate arrangement. It's an impromptu performance that vibrates through the hallways of the spirit, alleviating stress with its contagious and uplifting sounds.

In this symphony of relaxation techniques, beauty comes in their diversity. Individuals can curate their playlists, picking the strategies that resonate with their inner beat. Whether it's the tranquil cadence of deep breathing, the visual fabric of guided imagery, or the mindfulness meditation waltz, each approach allows individuals to build their own melody of relaxation, a timeless composition that harmonizes the mind, body, and spirit.

Importance of Quality Sleep in Diabetes Management

Imagine the nighttime stage as a sanctuary, where the curtains of darkness expose a performance important to the precise choreography of diabetes management. In this nocturnal play, sound sleep emerges as the unsung hero, assuming a cloak of regeneration and contributing to the vibrancy of the diabetic narrative.

The Nightly Rejuvenation Sonata opens with the conductor, melatonin, orchestrating the slow darkening of lights. This master signals the body to embrace a state of tranquility, setting the mood for the necessity of quality sleep. As the body enters the first movement, slow-wave sleep, it's akin to a quiet lullaby that cradles the mind and body in a restorative embrace.

Picture the second movement, the Rapid Eye Movement (REM) Allegro, as a spectacular excursion through the world of dreams. Here, the mind crafts stories, processes emotions, and consolidates memories. It's a strange dance that adds complexity to sleep composition, enhancing cognitive performance and emotional well-being.

With quality sleep, the virtuoso musician adjusts the hormonal symphony. The conductor cortisol takes a bow, enabling the crescendo of growth hormone and insulin to take center stage. This hormonal ensemble orchestrates the regeneration of cells, promotes tissue repair, and regulates glucose metabolism—a nocturnal ballet that harmonizes with the needs of diabetes care.

In the middle of this slumber serenade, the Stage of Blood Sugar Regulation appears as a vital stage piece. Here, the body navigates the delicate balance between insulin sensitivity and resistance. Quality sleep takes on the role of a professional choreographer, ensuring the dancer's blood sugar levels move in graceful harmony, preventing chaotic spikes and troughs.

As the Nightly Rejuvenation Sonata proceeds, the duet of Ghrelin and Leptin, hormones that govern hunger, delivers a mesmerizing routine. Quality sleep helps the dance by regulating these hormones, preventing the discordant notes of excessive appetite, and supporting a healthy weight—a critical factor in diabetes control.

The Symphony of Sleep extends its impact to the world of emotional resilience. Quality sleep functions as a guardian, protecting the mind against pressure and emotional instability. It's a nighttime shield that helps folks confront the challenges of diabetes management with renewed strength and mental clarity.

In the climactic crescendo, the Morning Awakening Overture, quality sleep graciously relinquishes its part, leaving the stage refreshed and rejuvenated. As the curtains fall on the Nightly Rejuvenation Sonata, the importance of quality sleep in the diabetes narrative becomes obvious. It's not only a nightly intermission; it's a cornerstone supporting the physical, mental, and metabolic elements of diabetes care. In this symphony of rest, the melody of sound sleep intertwines with the rhythm of well-being, creating a nocturnal masterpiece that resonates throughout the day.

Chapter 7

Holistic Approaches and Long-Term Strategies

Envision diabetes management as a dynamic symphony where holistic techniques and long-term tactics blend to create a timeless masterpiece. In this orchestration, the melody of complete well-being takes center stage, with each instrument playing a key role in preserving the rhythm of health.

Let's first comprehend the nuanced content of holistic nutrition, a movement that goes beyond simply nutrition. It's a culinary sonnet where nutrient-dense foods, rich in antioxidants and fiber, join forces to produce a harmony that nurtures the body. In this gastronomic symphony, the emphasis is not just on regulating blood sugar but also on boosting total energy.

As the nutrition movement grows, the rhythm of physical activity takes the limelight. Imagine a dance between the body and movement, a choreography that stretches beyond typical concepts of fitness. Whether it's a nature stroll, yoga, or a spirited dance, this movement transcends the limitations of a set regimen, becoming a joyful expression of health.

Picture the crescendo of stress management techniques, where awareness, deep breathing, and laughter intermingle. Stress, a subtle discordant note, is handled with a counter-harmony of relaxation practices. This movement acknowledges the psychological interplay in diabetes care, offering individuals the skills to build a tranquil mental landscape.

In the holistic symphony, the strings of social support and community engagement resound strongly. Imagine a network of humans, each performing a unique role in the song of support. It's a social composition where shared experiences, encouragement, and understanding become crucial in bolstering the emotional well-being of those navigating the diabetes path.

Now, let the brass section of regular monitoring and self-care practices take center stage. This movement is a vigilant guard, ensuring that blood sugar levels are not only detected but also responded to with proactive self-care. It's a robust melody that instills a sense of empowerment, changing mundane monitoring into a harmonious act of self-awareness.

As the holistic piece evolves, the woodwinds of mind-body techniques create an ethereal mood. Visualize activities like meditation and guided visualization weave through the mind, producing a tranquil ambiance that transcends the physical realm. This movement is a tribute to the delicate relationship between the mind and body, emphasizing the relevance of mental well-being in diabetes control.

In the final movement, the Percussion of Continuous Learning and Adaptation sets the rhythm. This is not a static composition but a dynamic symphony where individuals are lifelong learners, altering their techniques based on new insights and changing conditions. It's a dynamic cadence that represents the fluid essence of health.

In the grand finale, holistic approaches and long-term tactics blend into a symphony of health, where diabetes control is not a strict routine but a dynamic composition. It's a symphony that transcends the exclusive focus on blood sugar levels, embracing the complete well-being of the individual. As the curtain falls on this diabetes symphony, the resonance of holistic health lingers, allowing individuals to continue crafting their own harmonic narratives of well-being.

Mind-Body Practices for Diabetes

In the mosaic of diabetes management, the integration of mind-body activities appears as a significant brushstroke, constructing a narrative that transcends beyond the area of blood sugar control. These practices, profoundly based on ancient wisdom and modern science, unfold as a holistic canvas that addresses the subtle connection between mental well-being and physical health.

Consider the first stroke: the smooth pace of mindful meditation. Picture a tranquil lake where thoughts flow like soothing waves. In the field of diabetes, mindful meditation becomes a sanctuary where individuals acquire a non-judgmental awareness of their thoughts and feelings. It's a contemplative activity that offers a reprieve from the stresses of daily life, providing a mental space where tensions lose their grasp.

Now, visualize the brilliant hues of the Yoga Asana Palette. Beyond its physical postures, yoga becomes a mindful movement, a choreography of breath and body that transcends the constraints of a typical fitness regimen. This ancient technique increases flexibility, balance, and a profound sensation of inner serenity. In diabetes, yoga functions as a harmonious ally, supporting physical well-being while building mental resilience.

Next, explore the lovely melody of guided imagery. Picture a quiet scene—a sunlit meadow, a serene beach, or a thick forest. Guided imagery allows individuals to embark on a mental trip, transcending the boundaries of the current moment. In diabetes treatment, this technique becomes a therapeutic tapestry, a tool to alleviate stress and increase mental well-being.

As the canvas spreads, the rhythm of progressive muscle relaxation (PMR) takes center stage. Imagine a progressive release of tension, muscle by muscle, like unwinding a tightly coiled spring. PMR becomes a mindful dance, a practice that not only relaxes the physical body but also harmonizes with the psychological environment. In diabetes, where stress and tension can affect blood sugar levels, PMR emerges as a beneficial ally.

The picture of mind-body practices would be complete with the colorful strokes of breathwork. Visualize a rhythmic intake and exhalation, a dance of the breath that transcends its physiological function. Breathwork becomes a gateway to calmness, a technique someone can undertake anywhere, at any moment. In diabetes control, aware breathing becomes an accessible tool to traverse moments of stress and restore balance.

In the final strokes, the mosaic of mind-body practices forms a dynamic composition, offering individuals a palette of skills to enhance their general well-being. These practices give a chance to examine the significant connection between mental and physical health in the setting of diabetes care. As the brush leaves the painting, the beauty of mind-body activities continues to resonate—a song of awareness, movement, and calm that enhances the fabric of diabetes care.

Incorporating Meditation and Mindfulness

In the field of diabetes treatment, the art of incorporating meditation and mindfulness emerges as a transforming discipline, allowing individuals a sanctuary amidst the stresses of daily life. These contemplative approaches, anchored in ancient wisdom, become strong tools to navigate a complicated landscape of both bodily and mental well-being.

Imagine the practice of meditation as a calm excursion into the depths of the mind. Imagine a calm space—an undisturbed retreat where individuals can anchor themselves in the present moment. Meditation, in the context of diabetes, becomes a mental respite—an opportunity to disconnect from the concerns of blood sugar fluctuations and create a centered awareness.

In this meditative journey, mindfulness becomes a guiding light. Visualize the simple act of being present—a deliberate involvement with each moment without judgment. Mindfulness, analogous to a calm breeze, permits individuals to examine their thoughts and emotions without becoming entangled in them. This awareness extends to the arena of diabetes, creating a non-reactive approach toward the ever-changing panorama of blood sugar levels.

Consider the practice of mindful eating as a harmonious extension of this meditative approach. Picture a dining table where each meal becomes a purposeful act, savored with full attention. Conscious eating transforms meals into a conscious ceremony, enabling participants to appreciate the textures, flavors, and sustenance supplied by each morsel. In diabetes care, this exercise becomes a thoughtful dance with food, increasing both satisfaction and awareness of the body's response.

Now, consider the practice of body scan meditation as a delicate investigation of the physical self. Picture a gradual journey of attention from head to toe, a conscious release of tension from every muscle. Body Scan Meditation becomes a thoughtful dialogue with the body, offering a moment of self-compassion and relaxation. In the setting of diabetes, when stress can affect blood sugar levels, this practice becomes a vital ally in encouraging physical well-being.

As individuals adopt meditation and mindfulness into their diabetes care repertoire, these practices become a source of empowerment—a toolkit for navigating the ebb and flow of daily life with resilience. In the quiet moments of meditation and the purposeful presence in each breath, the art of mindfulness becomes a timeless companion on the journey of diabetes control. It's not only a practice; it's a gentle reminder that, amidst the complexity, the simplicity of the present moment may be a significant source of strength and well-being.

Yoga for Diabetes Wellness

In the area of diabetes wellness, the practice of yoga emerges as a gentle yet effective ally, offering a pathway to physical health and emotional stability. Visualize yoga not as an esoteric pursuit but as a basic and accessible tool that individuals may embrace on their road toward well-being.

Consider the practice of Yoga Asanas, or postures, as a set of moderate motions that can be tailored to varied fitness levels. These postures, typically inspired by nature and animals, enable individuals to explore the full range of motion in their bodies. From the stabilizing Mountain Pose to the calming Child's Pose, each asana becomes a thoughtful investigation of movement and breath.

Now, imagine the Breath-Centric Nature of yoga. Picture the rhythmic inhalations and exhalations that accompany each movement—a dance of breath and body. Yoga encourages individuals to connect breath with movement, creating not just a sensation of peace but also boosting the efficiency of the respiratory system. It becomes a thoughtful interaction between the body and the life-sustaining breath.

Imagine Yoga Nidra, or "yogic sleep," as a deep relaxation practice. Picture lying down, letting the body release tension progressively. In the context of diabetes management, where stress can affect blood sugar levels, Yoga Nidra becomes a beneficial method to induce relaxation, offering relief from the responsibilities of daily life.

In the simplicity of mindful meditation within yoga, individuals find a space for mental calm. Picture a peaceful time at the end of a yoga class, where the emphasis goes inward. This meditation becomes a conscious pause, allowing individuals to observe thoughts without judgment, generating a sense of mental clarity.

As individuals engage in yoga for diabetes wellness, they embark on a journey that surpasses the limitations of a standard workout program. Yoga becomes a partner, guiding folks toward physical flexibility, emotional resilience, and an enhanced feeling of general well-being. It's not about contorting into difficult postures but about embracing movement, breath, and mindfulness in a way that aligns with the unique rhythm of each individual. In the simplicity of yoga, individuals discover a pathway to balance—a comprehensive practice that goes beyond the mat, enriching their lives with the enduring blessings of health and vitality.

Mental Resilience and Diabetes

Mental resilience stands as a staunch partner, handling the trials with a steady attitude. The connection between the mind and diabetes is not only physiological; it's a sophisticated equilibrium that underlines the importance of mental well-being in the entire health equation.

Consider the daily practice of blood sugar monitoring, medication management, and lifestyle modifications. In this habit, mental resilience becomes a guiding force, helping individuals to endure the fluctuations with equanimity. It's not about removing the problems but rather growing the inner strength to respond with adaptation and composure.

Picture the role of a positive mindset in this equation. It's not a dismissal of the intricacies but a purposeful focus on potential. Individuals learn to reframe adversities as chances for progress, turning failures into stepping stones toward a better, more resilient self. A positive mindset becomes a lens through which individuals approach their diabetes journey, creating an optimistic view.

In the context of diabetes, where uncertainty can loom, stress management becomes a cornerstone of mental fortitude. Picture stress not as an inescapable element of life but as a passable terrain. Mindfulness practices, relaxation techniques, and the building of a supportive environment become tools to manage stress. These activities function as shields, protecting mental well-being amid the pressures of diabetes management.

Now, consider the concept of emotional intelligence as a compass leading individual through their emotional ups and downs. Recognizing and understanding emotions without judgment, individuals learn to respond wisely rather than react hastily. Emotional intelligence becomes a wellspring of strength, allowing individuals to handle the emotional intricacies of life with diabetes.

As individuals establish mental resilience, they are not only managing a medical problem; they are building a foundation for long-term well-being. It's not about eradicating the emotional nuances but rather embracing them with a resilience that converts problems into possibilities for growth. Mental resilience becomes a valuable ally, generating a sense of empowerment and self-efficacy on the diabetes path. In the simplicity of this resilience lies a tremendous power—a strength that enables individuals to not only manage diabetes but to thrive in the face of its complexity.

Chapter 8

Monitoring and Managing Blood Sugar Levels

Monitoring and regulating blood sugar levels constitute the cornerstone of good diabetes care, a practical and proactive strategy that empowers individuals in their day-to-day lives. It goes beyond the clinical sphere, involving a seamless integration of awareness, lifestyle modifications, and educated decision-making.

Routine Monitoring: At the basis of this approach lies routine monitoring. Individuals equipped with glucose meters or continuous glucose monitors smoothly incorporate these checks into their regular activities. It's a real-time examination providing insights into how the body responds to numerous elements like food, activity, and stress.

Nutritional Awareness: Consider nutritional choices as a dynamic element in blood sugar regulation. Individuals become builders of balanced meals, conscious of the glycemic impact of carbs, the significance of fiber, and the importance of portion control. It's about understanding food labels, making informed decisions, and arranging nutrition to maintain stable blood sugar levels.

Physical exercise integration: Physical exercise becomes a catalyst, not a chore. Engaging in workouts customized to individual tastes aids in insulin sensitivity and blood sugar stability. It's not about strenuous workouts but the rhythmic dance of movement—walking, cycling, or yoga—enhancing general well-being.

Medication Adherence: A vital issue requires adherence to prescribed drugs. Individuals create a disciplined practice, recognizing the timing, dose, and potential interactions. It's about aligning drug regimens with daily routines for seamless incorporation into life.

Proactive Decision-Making: In the dynamic flow of daily life, individuals make proactive decisions based on blood sugar levels. Adjusting insulin doses, opting for a nutritious snack, or modifying the workout routine—these options are responsive to the dynamic feedback supplied by blood sugar levels. It's a practical and inspiring strategy where individuals take responsibility for their health journey with informed decisions.

As the tale of blood sugar management unfolds, it's not a rigid control but a dynamic and flexible method. It's a journey where routine monitoring becomes a compass, leading individuals to navigate the complicated landscape of diabetes with knowledge, resilience, and a proactive spirit. Blood sugar management, under this method, transcends the numerical realm—it becomes a customized and empowered art of living well with diabetes.

Understanding Blood Glucose Monitoring

Understanding blood glucose monitoring is crucial to treating diabetes efficiently, giving individuals useful insights about their body's response to numerous stimuli. At its foundation, this approach entails regularly measuring the quantity of glucose in the bloodstream, offering real-time information vital for informed decision-making.

equipment of Monitoring: Blood glucose monitoring equipment, such as glucose meters and continuous glucose monitors (CGMs), are vital companions in this journey. These devices allow users to assess their blood sugar levels at several points throughout the day, producing a comprehensive picture of how their body responds to meals, physical exercise, and other variables.

Frequency and Timing: The frequency and timing of blood glucose measurements depend on individual circumstances and treatment strategies. For some, it might need routine monitoring before and after meals, while others may benefit from additional checks during the day. Consistent monitoring provides a clear insight into how dietary choices and everyday activities affect blood sugar levels.

Interpreting Readings: The numerical readings from blood glucose monitors are not just numbers—they are windows into the body's physiological processes. Individuals learn to interpret these readings in the context of their specific health profile. Understanding the goal range defined by healthcare professionals' aids individuals in analyzing whether their blood sugar levels are within the expected ranges.

Pattern identification: Monitoring blood glucose levels goes beyond isolated readings; it involves pattern identification. Individuals observe trends and variations, discovering patterns that assist them make intelligent adjustments to their lifestyle, medication, or nutritional choices. This proactive approach helps individuals to address potential concerns before they worsen.

Documentation and Analysis: Keeping a record of blood glucose measurements, combined with details about meals, activities, and medications, converts monitoring into a tailored analytical tool. This paperwork becomes a practical tool for healthcare professionals and individuals alike, supporting collaborative decision-making and modifications to the diabetes treatment strategy.

Emotional and Practical elements: Understanding blood glucose monitoring extends beyond the technical elements.

It entails acknowledging the emotional implications of managing a chronic condition. The habit of monitoring blood sugar becomes a real way for individuals to take charge of their health, generating a sense of empowerment in the face of diabetes.

In the simplicity of knowing blood glucose monitoring lies a significant strategy for efficient diabetes management. It's not just about statistics; it's about adopting a language—a dialogue with the body that helps individuals traverse the difficulties of diabetes with knowledge, precision, and a proactive attitude

Medication Management

Medication management is a cornerstone of diabetes treatment, reflecting a strategic alliance between individuals and healthcare professionals to improve health outcomes. It comprises a systematic approach to the administration, adherence, and adjustment of medications, ensuring that patients with diabetes attain and maintain stable blood sugar levels.

Precision in Dosage and Timing: At its core, drug management involves precision in dosage and timing. Individuals work closely with healthcare experts to identify the proper dosage of insulin or oral drugs depending on their specific health profile. Understanding the importance of adhering to recommended timetables enhances the efficacy of the treatment plan.

shared Decision-Making: Medication management is not a single undertaking but a shared adventure. Effective communication between individuals and healthcare professionals is vital. Open discussions regarding pharmaceutical experiences, anticipated side effects, and any problems faced enable modifications that correspond with individual needs and lifestyles.

Adherence as a Commitment: Adherence to the prescribed pharmaceutical regimen is a commitment to one's health. It goes beyond the act of taking medicines or delivering insulin—it shows an intentional decision to prioritize well-being. Regularly taking medications as advised assists greatly in obtaining and maintaining stable blood sugar levels.

Monitoring and Adjustments: Continuous monitoring of blood sugar levels plays a crucial role in drug management. Individuals track their responses to drugs, enabling timely modifications when necessary. This proactive approach helps individuals negotiate the changing nature of diabetes, making informed decisions to maximize their treatment strategy.

Integration into Daily living: Medication management is effortlessly interwoven into daily living. Whether it's carrying insulin pens, oral pills, or incorporating CGM devices, individuals make decisions that prioritize their health. The goal is to make medication a routine component of life, eliminating any hurdles to adherence.

Education as Empowerment: Understanding the purpose and mechanics of drugs is empowering. Individuals educated with knowledge about how medications operate, potential adverse effects and the necessity of adherence become active participants in their care. Education becomes a tool for educated decision-making.

In the simplicity of controlling drugs lies a great strategy for living well with diabetes. It's not only about pills and injections; it's about a dedication to health, a partnership with healthcare specialists, and a personalized strategy for managing the nuances of diabetes treatment. Medication management is a pragmatic and crucial component of the journey toward stable blood sugar levels and overall well-being.

Regular Health Checkups and Diabetes

Regular health checks are a cornerstone of proactive diabetes care, offering a key chance for individuals to evaluate their overall health and handle any issues. Beyond the normal monitoring of blood sugar levels, these exams serve as a full assessment of several areas of health, adding to a holistic approach to diabetes management.

Cardiovascular Health: Regular cardiovascular evaluations are necessary for patients with diabetes, given the heightened risk of heart-related problems. Monitoring blood pressure, and cholesterol levels, and assessing total heart function provide insights into the health of the cardiovascular system, allowing for early detection and management.

Kidney Function: Diabetes can influence kidney function over time. Regular checks include examinations of kidney health using tests that monitor kidney function and detect any signs of renal disease. Early diagnosis of possible concerns helps healthcare practitioners to implement treatments to protect renal function.

Eye Examinations: Diabetes can damage eyesight, making regular eye examinations vital. These examinations not only look for changes in vision but also test for diabetic retinopathy—a problem that can lead to vision impairment if left unchecked. Timely intervention can minimize the progression of eye-related problems.

Nerve Function: Nerve damage, known as neuropathy, is a typical consequence of diabetes. Regular health checkups may involve evaluations to examine nerve function, particularly in the extremities. Identifying indications of neuropathy enables preventative care to prevent additional consequences.

Foot Examinations: Foot health is crucial for patients with diabetes, as nerve damage and restricted blood circulation can lead to problems. Regular foot inspections assist spot any signs of injury, infection, or other conditions that could progress if not addressed soon. Preventive actions can then be implemented to preserve excellent foot health.

Weight Management: Monitoring weight and body mass index (BMI) is crucial to diabetes care. Regular checkups provide an opportunity to discuss and change weight management measures, ensuring that patients maintain a healthy weight to support overall well-being and blood sugar control.

Comprehensive Blood Tests: In addition to routine glucose monitoring, comprehensive blood tests are undertaken during health checks. These tests measure numerous markers, including HbA1c levels, offering a more extended perspective of blood sugar control over time. The results inform revisions to the diabetes management plan.

Regular health checkups, therefore, go beyond basic inspections; they exemplify a proactive and preventive approach to diabetes care. By addressing possible issues early on, individuals can work cooperatively with healthcare experts to personalize their treatment plans, guaranteeing a balanced and comprehensive strategy for overall health and well-being.

Chapter 9

Crafting Your Ongoing Action Plan

Crafting your continuous action plan for diabetes management is a dynamic process that incorporates numerous parts of your daily life into a cohesive strategy for optimal well-being. This tailored plan changes over time, according to your specific requirements, experiences, and changing health circumstances.

Reflecting on your own objectives: Begin by reflecting on your own objectives. What parts of your life and health do you wish to prioritize? Whether it's reaching stable blood sugar levels, keeping a healthy weight, or preventing complications, defining your objectives forms the foundation of your action plan.

adapting Lifestyle Choices: Your continuous action plan entails adapting lifestyle choices to meet with your health goals. This comprises food preferences, physical activity levels, and stress management measures. Integrating these decisions into your routine ensures that they become durable and supportive of your diabetes control.

Adapting Physical Exercise: Regular physical exercise is crucial to diabetes control. Craft an action plan that incorporates exercises you enjoy and that fit easily into your regular routine. Whether it's walking, riding, or indulging in other forms of exercise, choosing activities that bring fulfillment boosts adherence.

Fine-Tuning Dietary Habits: Your continuous action plan should address dietary habits, stressing a balanced and diabetes-friendly approach. Work with healthcare specialists to understand the influence of different foods on your blood sugar levels and make informed decisions that match with your nutritional needs.

Continual monitoring and modifications: Embrace an attitude of continual monitoring and modifications. Regularly check your blood sugar levels, adhere to prescribed medications, and assess the influence of lifestyle choices. This proactive approach enables you to make timely adjustments to your strategy, ensuring it remains effective in achieving your health goals.

Prioritizing Mental and Emotional Well-being: Crafting a successful action plan entails prioritizing mental and emotional well-being. Incorporate stress management practices, such as mindfulness and relaxation exercises, into your regimen. Building resilience and managing emotional issues are key components of a holistic approach.

Building a Support System: Recognize the necessity of a support system. Whether it's family, friends, or healthcare experts, incorporate those who can contribute positively to your journey. Effective communication ensures that your support system understands your goals and can provide encouragement and assistance as needed.

Regular Health Checkups: Integrate regular health checkups into your continuing action plan. These examinations serve as a proactive tool to examine your overall health, monitor potential issues, and fine-tune your management measures based on professional advice.

Crafting your ongoing action plan is not a static undertaking; it's a constant process of modification and adaptation. By evaluating the specific factors of your life, setting realistic goals, and keeping open to revisions, you develop a dynamic framework that helps you handle the intricacies of diabetes management with confidence and resilience.

Reflecting on Progress

In the continual journey of treating diabetes, the practice of reflecting on progress acts as a vital compass, guiding individuals through the intricate landscape of their health and well-being. This introspective exercise extends beyond only checking blood sugar levels; it covers a complete review of lifestyle choices, emotional well-being, and the dynamics of personal support systems.

Celebrating triumphs becomes a cornerstone of this reflection, motivating individuals to acknowledge and praise even the tiniest victories in their diabetes control. These milestones may range from effectively incorporating healthy food habits to regularly adhering to prescribed medications. The act of celebration cultivates a positive mindset, producing a sense of accomplishment that motivates individuals ahead on their health path.

A major component of this reflection entails examining blood sugar control with a careful eye. Examining patterns and trends helps individuals discover the impact of their everyday choices on glucose levels. Understanding the connection between nutrition, physical exercise, and pharmaceuticals helps individuals to adapt their approach, assuring more effective management.

Beyond the sphere of physiological measures, the examination extends to lifestyle adjustments. Consideration is given to adjustments in food choices, the incorporation of physical exercise, and the adoption of stress management approaches. Reflecting on these improvements allows individuals to identify their impact on overall well-being and suggests adjustments when needed.

Challenges, considered not as setbacks but as chances for learning, are acknowledged in this reflective process. By exploring the core reasons for setbacks, individuals obtain insights into triggers and impediments that may hamper progress. This self-awareness becomes a driver for generating targeted tactics to overcome problems and reinforce resilience.

Emotional well-being emerges as a significant factor in this reflective journey. Recognizing the impact of stress, anxiety, and other emotions on diabetes management motivates the inclusion of mindfulness and self-care activities. Addressing emotional health helps to a more complete and sustainable approach to overall well-being.

The evaluation also goes to the robustness of one's support system. The roles of family, friends, and healthcare professionals are explored, with open communication and teamwork being crucial components. This contemplation motivates individuals to develop and strengthen their support networks, acknowledging their vital role in the diabetes control journey.

Setting realistic goals and reassessing them in light of developing circumstances is another part of this introspective activity. Goals that are aligned with an individual's aspirations and flexible to changing health priorities stay inspiring and contribute to long-term success.

Continuous education becomes a vital element of this introspective path. Staying educated on the latest breakthroughs in diabetes treatment helps that individuals make decisions based on the most up-to-date knowledge. This commitment to learning helps individuals to navigate their health journey with informed decisions.

Looking forward, this introspective process becomes a tool for thoughtful planning. It supports individuals in making improvements to their diabetes care plan based on insights gathered. Establishing realistic short-term and long-term goals becomes a forward-looking exercise that maintains alignment with an individual's overall health desires.

Reflecting on progress in controlling diabetes is not a solitary event but an ongoing process. It is a conscious and informed attitude that appreciates achievements, learns from problems, and makes intentional choices for a future that prioritizes health and well-being.

Adjusting Your Lifestyle for Long-Term Success

With the aim of controlling diabetes for long-term success, the adjustment of one's lifestyle emerges as a vital and dynamic process. This transformation requires intentional adaptations that transcend beyond temporary changes, promoting habits and choices that become embedded in daily life. It is a progression, guided by a commitment to health and well-being, and it embraces various parts of an individual's life.

Dietary modifications play a crucial role in this transforming journey. Rather than viewing dietary changes as restrictive measures, individuals are taught to see them as a gateway to fueling their bodies optimally. Embracing a balanced and diabetes-friendly diet becomes not only a short-term adjustment but a sustained lifestyle decision. This requires learning the intricacies of portion control, choosing nutrient-dense meals, and navigating the glycemic index to make smart dietary selections.

Physical activity, typically viewed as a cornerstone of a healthy lifestyle, takes center stage in the pursuit of long-term success in diabetes control. The goal is not merely to engage in irregular exercise but to weave physical activity smoothly into the fabric of daily life. This may mean choosing pleasurable activities, whether it's walking, cycling, or engaging in formal fitness regimens, building a love for movement that endures over time.

Stress management plays a crucial part in this lifestyle transition. Recognizing stress as a possible disruptor in diabetes control drives individuals to study and use effective stress reduction measures. Whether through mindfulness practices, relaxation techniques, or hobbies that provide joy, stress management becomes a vital aspect of preserving long-term well-being.

Sleep, frequently underappreciated in its impact on health, is brought into focus during this lifestyle shift. Prioritizing excellent sleep and appreciating its enormous influence on blood sugar levels and general health becomes a non-negotiable component. Creating a suitable sleep environment and establishing consistent sleep habits contribute to a comprehensive approach to diabetes care.

Social ties and relationships are regarded as crucial pillars in this journey. Recognizing the effect of a solid support system on mental and emotional well-being, individuals are urged to build ties with family, friends, and the diabetic community. Building a robust support network becomes an enduring component of the lifestyle shift, providing encouragement and understanding throughout both accomplishments and setbacks.

Regular monitoring and checkups become typical components of this altered lifestyle. Rather than considering them as occasional tasks, individuals appreciate the proactive role of regular health exams. This continual commitment to monitoring blood sugar levels, health markers, and overall well-being serves as a preventive and empowering approach to the long-term management of diabetes.

Crucially, this lifestyle shift reframes the narrative around diabetes management. It transforms the focus from a succession of discrete activities to a complete and integrated strategy that tackles the interconnection of physical, emotional, and mental well-being. It encourages individuals to view their health journey as an ongoing investment, with each change adding to the sustainable success of controlling diabetes over the long run.

Modifying one's lifestyle for long-term success in diabetes control is a conscious and constant process of refining. It is not a drastic departure from the familiar but a planned adaptation that corresponds with the objective of nurturing permanent health and well-being. This method develops a sense of empowerment, resilience, and a consistent commitment to a lifestyle that supports individuals on their journey toward sustained success in treating diabetes.

Building a Sustainable Future Without Diabetes

As we envision a future free from the limits of diabetes, the focus changes toward establishing a sustainable and health-centric existence. This endeavor beyond the management of symptoms; it is a proactive and holistic approach aimed at promoting a life where the burden of diabetes is reduced, if not removed totally.

At the heart of this vision is the commitment to a lifestyle that fosters health and well-being. This lifestyle is not a temporary adjustment but a lasting foundation built on informed decisions and aware habits. Central to this approach is the awareness and inclusion of balanced nutrition, where food choices become a source of sustenance rather than restriction.

Physical activity, seen as a vital element of a healthy existence, takes precedence in crafting a future without diabetes. The idea is not only to engage in irregular exercise but to integrate movement effortlessly into daily routines. This means finding delight in physical activity, embracing a varied range of workouts, and building a real awareness of the positive influence of movement on overall health.

In this envisioned future, stress is acknowledged as a possible disruptor of well-being. Stress management tactics become integrated into daily life, with individuals investigating and adopting practices that bring about relaxation and mental equilibrium. The goal is to cultivate a resilient mindset capable of facing life's obstacles without compromising health.

Sleep, acknowledged for its tremendous influence on health, becomes a cornerstone of this sustainable future. Prioritizing and optimizing sleep patterns are key components of the vision, and understanding the importance quality sleep plays in metabolic balance and general vitality.

The creation of a robust support system represents a crucial part of this future without diabetes. Relationships with family, friends, and the broader community become a source of support, understanding, and shared experiences. The diabetes community, in particular, emerges as a vital resource for mutual support and shared insights.

Regular monitoring of health markers and preventive exams become engrained behaviors, not as reactionary measures but as proactive efforts toward preserving good health. This dedication to periodic health assessments serves as a preventive strategy, allowing for early intervention and adjustment as needed.

Constructing a sustainable future without diabetes is a dynamic and continuing process. It is a dedication to a lifestyle that emphasizes health, adopts preventative measures, and continuously adjusts to evolving conditions. This future is not determined by the absence of obstacles but by the resilience and drive to handle them while safeguarding well-being.

In this envisioned future, humans are not only treating diabetes; they are actively constructing a life that surpasses the limits often associated with the condition. It is a future where health is not a compromise but a persistent commitment, and the journey toward a sustainable, diabetes-free existence becomes a tribute to the power of educated choices, resilience, and the unflinching pursuit of optimal well-being.

Conclusion

In ending our research into the diverse domain of diabetes treatment and lifestyle transformation, it is crucial to highlight the pivotal role that educated decisions and proactive measures play in supporting long-term well-being. This journey has been more than an examination of managing a medical condition; it has been an invitation to embrace a lifestyle that surpasses the constraints generally associated with diabetes.

The information gained throughout this thorough guide goes beyond the nuances of blood sugar levels and medication management; it stretches to the very fabric of our daily lives. It emphasizes the power of lifestyle alterations, nutrition choices, and the importance of an active and healthy existence in minimizing the burden of diabetes.

Crucially, our journey together has spotlighted the need for a proactive approach to health. It is not only about reacting to symptoms or according to a set of rules; it is about embracing an attitude that places health at the center of our priorities. The commitment to regular health checks, blood glucose monitoring, and a consistent endeavor towards a diabetes-friendly lifestyle provides the core of this proactive posture.

In essence, this handbook acts as a compass, pointing towards a future where the story of diabetes is not one of restriction but of empowerment. It underlines the possibility for individuals to take care of their health, make choices that nourish the body and mind, and develop a sustainable and resilient lifestyle that extends far beyond the management of a medical condition.

As we draw this trip to an end, it is with the goal that the ideas imparted will not only enlighten but inspire. The path to diabetes-friendly living is not a strict formula; it is a dynamic and ongoing adventure. It is a path distinguished by the empowerment to make choices aligned with health and vitality, ultimately leading to a future where the impact of diabetes is minimized, and the quest for well-being becomes a rewarding and enduring activity.

Celebrating Successes and Milestones

In the journey towards managing diabetes, recognizing victories and milestones becomes a vital aspect of maintaining a positive and resilient mindset. Each step taken, every milestone attained, and every positive adjustment made in one's lifestyle deserves praise and celebration. It is in recognizing and celebrating these wins that individuals find the desire and inspiration to stay on the path to a better and more satisfying life.

Acknowledging and celebrating triumphs is not just about accomplishing specific health goals; it is also about acknowledging the commitment, discipline, and determination that go into making those achievements possible. Whether it's maintaining constant blood sugar levels, adopting a more diabetes-friendly diet, or adding regular exercise to daily activities, each small accomplishment contributes to the greater narrative of well-being.

These celebrations act as potent reinforcement, reinforcing the belief that positive change is not only attainable but also within reach. They offer individuals with a sense of accomplishment, enhancing self-esteem and confidence in their ability to navigate the intricacies of diabetes care. More than just markers of progress, these milestones become beacons of hope and resilience.

Moreover, celebrating victories produces a positive feedback loop, encouraging individuals to continue engaged in their health path. It instills a mindset that perceives setbacks as chances for progress rather than insurmountable hurdles. By reflecting on and appreciating victories, individuals create a mindset that encourages long-term commitment to a diabetes-friendly lifestyle.

The act of celebration is a recognition of the continual work placed on personal wellness. It is a chance to pause, reflect, and celebrate the strides achieved towards a better and more vibrant existence. Whether it's a modest acknowledgment of personal triumphs or sharing successes with a support system, these celebrations contribute greatly to the emotional and psychological well-being of those managing diabetes. In the big time of life, each celebration becomes a colorful thread, weaving a narrative of triumph over trials and fortitude in the face of adversity.

Empowered and Diabetes-Free: Your Journey Ahead

Embarking on the journey towards empowerment and a life free from the constraints of diabetes is a profound and deeply personal endeavor. It is a journey that transcends the boundaries of health and extends into the realm of self-discovery and personal transformation. As individuals navigate the path ahead, they find themselves equipped with newfound knowledge, resilience, and a sense of agency over their well-being.

Central to this journey is the understanding that empowerment in diabetes management is not merely about controlling blood sugar levels but involves a holistic transformation of lifestyle and mindset. It encompasses a commitment to making informed choices, embracing a health-conscious diet, and incorporating regular physical activity as an integral component of daily life.

Empowerment, in the context of diabetes, is rooted in the belief that individuals can shape their health destiny. It is about taking ownership of one's well-being, making decisions that align with long-term health goals, and understanding that each choice, no matter how small, contributes to the larger picture of a diabetes-free life.

The journey ahead involves cultivating a mindset that views challenges as opportunities for growth and learning. It is about resilience in the face of setbacks, adaptability to evolving circumstances, and a continuous pursuit of knowledge to refine and optimize the approach to diabetes management.

As individuals progress on this empowering journey, they not only witness improvements in physical health but also experience a profound shift in their mental and emotional well-being. There is a sense of liberation that comes from breaking free from the shackles of a condition that once seemed insurmountable. It is about living with intention, purpose, and the unwavering belief that a diabetes-free life is not just an aspiration but an achievable reality.

Furthermore, the journey towards empowerment is not a solitary endeavor. It thrives on the support of healthcare professionals, family, and friends who provide encouragement, understanding, and a network of support. Building and nurturing these connections becomes an integral part of the path forward, creating a robust foundation for sustained well-being.

In conclusion, the road to an empowered and diabetes-free life is a transformative and liberating expedition. It is a journey that unfolds with each conscious choice, each healthy meal, and each step taken toward a more active and fulfilling life. As individuals navigate this path, they discover the profound strength that resides within them, paving the way for a future that is not defined by diabetes but empowered by the choices made today.

Diabetes-Friendly Recipes

On a journey towards managing diabetes entails not just knowing the condition but also adopting a lifestyle that supports health and well-being. Central to this lifestyle is a balanced and nutritious diet, and what better way to embrace this than through a variety of tasty and diabetes-friendly recipes?

These recipes are meticulously developed to establish a healthy balance between taste and health, guaranteeing that those with diabetes can enjoy a varied range of delectable meals without compromising their well-being. The emphasis is on combining nutrient-dense nutrients that contribute to stable blood sugar levels.

Consider recipes that incorporate lean proteins like grilled chicken or fish, accompanied by an array of vibrant veggies. These not only bring vibrancy to your plate but also supply critical vitamins and minerals. Whole grains, such as quinoa or brown rice, can replace processed carbohydrates, delivering a more consistent flow of energy.

For those with a sweet craving, there are imaginative dessert options that rely on natural sweeteners or alternatives to regular sugar. Think of desserts that showcase the natural sweetness of fruits or experiment with sugar substitutes to create guilt-free delights.

Moreover, these recipes are not simply about restriction but about culinary experimentation. They encourage the use of herbs and spices to heighten flavors without the need for excessive salt or sugar. The idea is to transform every meal into a joyful experience while keeping a diabetes-friendly approach.

Incorporating these recipes into your routine isn't just about managing diabetes; it's about savoring each mouthful, appreciating the different flavors on your plate, and embracing a lifestyle that nurtures both your palette and your well-being. So, let these recipes be your guide to a culinary experience that's not just excellent for your health but also a joy for your taste senses.

Fitness Routine Samples

On a fitness journey is a serious commitment to one's total well-being, and developing a routine that corresponds with individual goals and preferences is vital to its durability. Here, we study samples of workout routines tailored to accommodate diverse fitness levels and tastes.

For individuals going into the world of fitness or returning after a hiatus, a beginner's regimen could comprise a mix of aerobic exercises like brisk walking or cycling, complimented by bodyweight exercises such as squats, lunges, and push-ups. The emphasis here is on developing a firm foundation and progressively increasing intensity.

Intermediate fitness lovers might find a combination of cardio and strength training ideal. This could involve activities like jogging, swimming, or cycling, combined with resistance training utilizing weights or resistance bands. The idea is to boost the heart rate while progressively taxing the muscles for better strength and endurance.

Advanced exercise routines are geared toward people desiring a higher level of difficulty. High-intensity interval training (HIIT) sessions, involving explosive movements and complicated exercises, can push the frontiers of cardiovascular fitness and strength. Activities like CrossFit or advanced weightlifting regimens fit within this group.

For those with special exercise goals such as flexibility or stress reduction, programs like yoga or Pilates can be implemented. These not only contribute to bodily well-being but also build mental resilience and calm.

The secret to a great exercise routine resides in variety and improvement. Mixing up activities not only keeps things interesting but also guarantees that different muscle areas are utilized, minimizing monotony and potential overuse problems.

It's crucial to listen to your body, allowing for rest and healing as needed. A well-rounded fitness regimen should be sustainable and pleasurable, developing a good relationship with exercise rather than perceiving it as a mere obligation.

These fitness routine samples are mere templates. Tailoring them to individual interests, fitness levels, and goals is the secret to a lifetime dedication to health and fitness. Whether it's the simplicity of a brisk walk or the intensity of a high-intensity workout, the trip towards fitness is a personal quest, and finding what works for you is key.

Additional Resources for Continued Learning

In the pursuit of knowledge about diabetes treatment and general well-being, accessing extra resources for continuing learning is a valuable step. These resources extend beyond the primary material presented and offer varied perspectives, in-depth insights, and continuous support.

One key resource is renowned health organizations, such as the American Diabetes Association and the World Health Organization. Their websites often include a plethora of information, including articles, guidelines, and tools, providing a solid foundation for understanding diabetes and its care.

Medical periodicals and publications are vital for people who want to stay updated on the newest research and breakthroughs in diabetes care. Peer-reviewed articles and scientific studies offer a deeper grasp of developing trends, treatment approaches, and developments in the field.

Online courses and webinars can be beneficial for anyone seeking structured instruction. Many educational platforms provide courses on nutrition, fitness, and diabetes care, providing interactive and interesting content that caters to diverse learning styles.

Support groups and forums give a sense of community for individuals confronting similar issues. Connecting with others who share experiences and thoughts develops a supportive environment. Organizations like Diabetes Daily or local community groups may give these possibilities for contact.

Health apps and digital solutions customized for diabetes management provide real aid. From tracking blood sugar levels to delivering individualized nutrition advice, these gadgets can be helpful companions on the journey towards optimal health.

Books produced by healthcare experts or persons with knowledge in diabetes management can provide varied viewpoints. Personal narratives and expert insights, frequently found in well-researched books, can give practical recommendations and motivation.

Podcasts on diabetes health and well-being are gaining popularity. Listening to professionals, clinicians, and individuals discussing their experiences can be an accessible and entertaining way to stay informed while on the road.

In conclusion, the pursuit of knowledge doesn't cease with the last chapter of a book. Engaging with extra resources, from authoritative websites to supportive groups and digital tools, deepens the learning experience and empowers individuals on their continued journey towards a healthier, more informed existence.